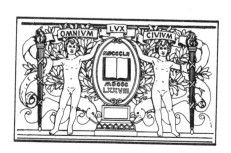

Cognitive Science Series, 8

Eric Wanner, General Editor

Advisory Board

Cognitive Science Series

Language
and Experience

Evidence from the Blind Child

Barbara Landau and
Lila R. Gleitman

Harvard University Press
Cambridge, Massachusetts
London, England
1985

Printed in the United States of America

10 9 8 7 6 5 4 3 2 1

This book is printed on acid-free paper, and
its binding materials have been chosen for
strength and durability.

Library of Congress Cataloging in Publication Data

Landau, Barbara, 1949–
    Language and experience.

    (Cognitive science series; 8)
    Bibliography: p.
    Includes index.
    1. Language acquisition. 2. Children, Blind—
Language. I. Gleitman, Lila R. II. Title. III. Series.
P118.L24 1985   401′.9   85-783
ISBN 0-674-51025-9 (alk. paper)

To our parents

Nora and Manuel
Fanny and Ben

Preface

We ask in this book how children learn which of the words in their language encode which of the meanings. We accept as self-evident that any explanation of this learning must take nonlinguistic experience as relevant: When children hear words spoken by adults, they also observe objects, scenes, and events. Yet the issues here are quite perplexing because, at least to first inspection, heard words seem to map only very inexactly onto the child's observations of objects, scenes, and events. After all, it must with some frequency be the case that the child learner is attending to one thing (say, the ice cream on the sideboard) while the mother speaks of something else ("Eat your peas, dear!"). Woe to the learner who takes this particular word-to-experience pair as a basis for reconstructing the meanings conveyed by language.

In light of such difficulties, we tried to get some insight into how the child constructs the right mappings between words and the world by examining a situation in which the opportunities to observe the world are diminished: the case of language learning by congenitally blind children. This approach is hardly new. Such philosophers as Locke and Leibniz considered the case of the congenitally blind to be crucial to their epistemological theories. From Locke's perspective, it was clear that the blind should be defective in their understanding of certain words, such as *picture* or *blue*, for he held that the concepts they encode can be derived only from specific sensory experience. In contrast, Liebniz held that much of this knowledge arises internally, and is not dependent on the information afforded by the individual senses—that in the end, "the geometries of the blind man and the paralytic must come together and agree."

We have tried to study blind children in a way that might be pertinent to this debate. To do so, we first studied the milestones in three blind children's acquisition of English speech. And we studied the comprehension of word meaning as this emerged in one blind subject during the first six years of her life. In particular, we asked about the meanings of vision-related terms such as *look* and *color*, for these items represent the case in which the experiences of the blind child and the sighted child appear to be maximally different. The outcomes of these investigations are most naturally interpreted as showing that the blind learner can surmount whatever obstacles the diminution of experience places in her path, acquiring her native tongue in a largely unexceptional fashion. As we will show, this success extends to comprehension of the vision-related terms. Our main purpose has been to try to discuss these findings as they bear on the general problem of induction which all children—blind and sighted—confront in acquiring their native tongue.

At the extremes, there are two ways of thinking about the blind child's linguistic competence. One is to suppose that the role of experience as the causal force in language acquisition is more restricted than common sense would lead one to suppose. The other is that, under an appropriate analysis of experience, the blind child's situation is not as abnormal or deprived as common sense would lead one to suppose. These approaches are not mutually contradictory, and we will have to advance explanations in terms of each of them to understand aspects of what our subjects came to know. Nonetheless, at bottom ours is chiefly an experience-based approach to the child's discovery of his native tongue. To maintain this view in face of the blind child's manifest competence, we draw heavily on the idea that while much of the learner's relevant experience comes from observation of the situational concomitants of the speech he hears, crucial further observations implicated in his solution to the linguistic puzzle are of language structure itself.

The findings reported herein, as well as their interpretations, stand in direct opposition to claims about language learning that appear in the current literature. There is an evidently unshakable tradition which asserts that the blind must in principle be defective in their learning—of language, of space, and more. So powerful are these beliefs that they are often asserted with confidence, without thought of conducting investigation to show whether or not they are true. Thus clinicians advise parents of blind children to touch the children's legs six times a day to give the tots an idea of space (which they could not have "because" they are blind) and—more to the issues taken up in this book—to prohibit the children from saying such things as "I see" (which they could not understand "because" they are blind). One might guess that such presuppositions without evidentiary basis would be restricted to clinical practitioners who work outside the scientific tradition. But unfortunately this is not so. Even scientists whose professional concern it is to develop empirical evidence on the problem of language learning are quite willing to assert the facts about blind learners without investigating them at all. For example, Lois Bloom commented with puzzling confidence in a recent issue of *Science* that blind children's language must be "disjoint in meaning" and "distorted" because these children are deprived of "input from the context." And recently Paul Werth, commenting in a scholarly volume on one of the very children whose competence we will document herein—and presenting no evidence whatsoever—remarked, "The sad fact is that the language of Kelli and children like her is *inevitably* deficient" to the extent that "for blind people there is an area of experience which can never be detailed at first hand."

We shall document that these *a priori* opinions cannot survive confrontation with the reality of language learning in congenitally blind children. Blind learners not only learn the forms of language but their meanings as well; their speech cannot be characterized as replete with "verbalisms" (the clinical term for blind learners' putative use of certain words as "sound without meaning"). Perhaps our deepest aim is to understand why both clinicians and developmental psychologists believe they know the facts here in advance, why evidence is not taken to be relevant. In our view, these commentators and practitioners can be most sympathetically understood as motivated by a coherent philosophical persuasion close to the more extreme versions of British empiricism: All knowledge begins with, and its character is a straightforward derivative of, the raw discriminations of the sensory apparatus; if that apparatus is defective, so must be the knowledge. We believe that the findings presented herein—though, to be sure, they are partial and fragmentary in many ways—support the view that this is merely one epistemological hypothesis among many plausible ones, and perhaps not the easiest to defend as an account of the language-learning feat.

In beginning, we wish to express our gratitude to the many who have helped us to think and write about these issues.

First we extend our warmest thanks to the young blind child, Kelli. Before we began any "experiments," she made clear to us through the intelligence and spark of her everyday acts and speech that the young blind child is just a child who happens not to be able to see, not a person with special cognitive or linguistic

"deficits." Kelli's mother, too, made clear to us from the beginning that she considered her blind child to be fully functioning
rather than especially handicapped in speech or cognitive development; this point of view, quite different from that of the pro-
fessionals we have mentioned above, led her to join us in discovering the depth and breadth of Kelli's knowledge. Many of the
specific experiments we will report were motivated by this
mother's anecdotes about Kelli, which we then documented more
formally.

We wish to thank a number of colleagues without whose help
we could never have understood our findings or expressed them
in anything like the way we have done. Two colleagues were involved with the project from start to finish and their influence appears throughout the manuscript. Henry Gleitman helped us in
the conception and development of the study, constantly forcing
us to think about whether we were studying language or perception (or both); thereafter he worked with us almost line by line
and crisis by crisis, challenging our claims and assumptions, contributing materially to the substance and ideas in terms of which
the findings are organized and presented, and even descending to
the level of correcting our grammar and spelling. Eric Wanner
originally encouraged us to write up the findings as a book that
emphasized the induction problem in language learning. He then
read and reread many versions of this manuscript, supplying new
and clarifying ideas both about the theoretical claims we made
and about the presentation of findings; in addition, he acted as the
formal editor for the book, we think very effectively. We cannot
thank these two individuals strongly enough or often enough.

We also extend our thanks to Noam Chomsky who (along with
Henry Gleitman) encouraged us to investigate and discuss the
maternal input to the blind child much more seriously than we
had thought to do—to ask, finally, *how* the blind child learned
what she did; to Elizabeth Shipley, who helped us to deepen the
discussion of constraints on lexical concepts; to Elizabeth Spelke,
who helped us think about the distinction between knowledge
and perception, and what the blind child's understanding of visual verbs implied about this problem; and to Scott Weinstein,
who coaxed us to discuss the findings from the perspective of philosophy and helped us decide how to do so. Each of the people
just mentioned also aided us by patiently reading successive versions of this manuscript, offering extremely helpful discussions
and ideas each time through it.

We had the advantage of readings of earlier drafts and critical
reviews and discussions from a number of other individuals to

whom we express our gratitude here. These are Tom Bever, Julian Hochberg, Ray Jackendoff, Jerry Fodor, Janet Levin, Elissa Newport, Dan Osherson, Ruth Ostrin, Sudan Scanlon, and Ken Wexler. Further colleagues to whom we extend thanks for very helpful discussions are Rochel Gelman, Jane Grimshaw, Dick Neisser, Ed Pugh, and Stan Peters.

We also thank the physicians and social workers who first identified our subjects for us, and who continued to retain an active interest in the work as it proceeded: Dr. Judy Bernbaum, Anne Farren, and Dr. Gilberto Pereira. Our research assistants helped us carry out this work and contributed substantive ideas as well. These were Anne Edwards, Kathy Feldman, Claire Gleitman, Marcia Glicksman, Sharon Kessler, Lenora Knapp, and Mark Schneider. Many thanks to Rob Thacker for going out of his way to do such an extraordinary job with the drawings. Thanks also go to Annette Hartstein, our administrative assistant, who aided significantly with stylistic matters and facilitated preparation of the manuscript in very important ways. Robert Landau provided crucial personal support, as well as our new shoes with matching handbags.

Three granting agencies provided the funding for this work, and we thank them for their support: A National Foundation–March of Dimes Social and Behavioral Sciences Research Grant provided the major funding for the work; a predoctoral award to Barbara Landau from the National Institutes of Mental Health and a postdoctoral award to her from the Alfred P. Sloan Foundation also were of material aid.

Most of all we thank the parents and the children who served as the subjects and participants in this work and who, with constant humor, warmth, and patience, allowed us to understand the blind child's experience, and to become their friends.

B.L.
L.G.

Philadelphia, December 1984

Contents

Language and Experience

Evidence from the Blind Child

1 / Language and Experience

If we will observe how children learn languages,
we shall find that, to make them understand what
the names of simple ideas or substances stand
for, people ordinarily show them the thing
whereof they would have them have the idea; and
then repeat to them the name that stands for it,
as 'white', 'sweet', 'milk', 'sugar', 'cat', 'dog'.

(John Locke, 1690, Book 3.IX.9)

To know a language is to know the relations between sounds and their meanings. Since these relations vary over the languages of the world—in English /si/ means 'gaze with the eyes' but in Spanish /si/ means 'yes'—it follows that the child must acquire them by induction from specific experience. Common sense requires us to agree with Locke that the relevant inductions have to do with ascertaining how heard speech relates to objects, scenes, and events the learner is experiencing as he listens. After all, how could it be otherwise? If you saw rhinoceroses when we said "giraffes," you might learn a language, but it wouldn't be *our* language. All parties who have thought about language learning—from the early empiricists such as Locke and Berkeley to rationalists such as Leibniz, and from behaviorists such as Bloomfield (1933) and sociocommunicative theorists such as Bruner (1974–75) to learnability theorists such as Wexler and Culicover (1980)—agree thus far: Some interpretive context, paired with speech events, is required if language learning is to get off the ground floor.

No disagreement arises, then, about the *necessity* for extralinguistic experience. But despite this agreement, the theorists just mentioned vary considerably in their conceptions of how language is attained by the young child. Their disagreements have to do with the *sufficiency* of experience for learning a language. Exactly how is the relevant external experience to be internally represented? How could anyone *use* this experience to learn a language? How could seeing a dog while hearing "dog" determine that /dɔg/ means 'dog'?[1]

In this book, we take up the case of language learning by blind children. This topic seems relevant to questions about the role of experience in language learning because, at least on first inspection, the blind seem to confront a world quite different from our own. To the extent that blind children's extralinguistic contexts for the words and sentences they hear differ from those of sighted children, one might expect their language learning to differ as well. And to the extent that learning really does differ, the role of experience in building a mental lexicon may be clarified. This is because the problem of language learning for any individual, however circumstanced, is a problem of learning from partial information. No one requires experience of every dog to acquire the word *dog*. It is this strikingly uniform acquisition of language, based on only partial and sometimes quite impoverished relevant experiences, that makes a mystery of language induction. We expect to gain insight into the nature of this problem by examining language learning in the blind child, who evidently must work with a different inductive base.

In our studies we focussed on three questions about how experiential deprivations might affect blind children:

(1) Is their language acquisition seriously delayed or grossly distorted because of limits on available contextual support?

(2) Are their difficulties centered on linguistic items and structures that, for sighted people, describe visible things or the visual experience?

(3) Is their learning, to the extent that it is successful, a consequence of special adjustments made by their sighted caregivers?

To address the first question, we studied the standard milestones in three blind children's acquisition of a first language, comparing these with accounts in the literature for sighted children. Both for syntax and for word learning, extreme differences in what is learned early and easily by blind and sighted children might be expected, assuming that extralinguistic experience is the driving causal force in language learning. Oddly enough, our general finding is that the blind children develop much as do their sighted agemates.

To approach the second question, we investigated in detail a blind child's development for two apparently sight-related categories: her use and interpretation of the verbs *look* and *see* (as compared to aural and tactual verbs such as *hear* and *touch*) and her use and interpretation of the adjectives of color (*red* and *green* as opposed to other property terms such as *big* and *round*). Surely if extralinguistic experience provides the route to learning, a blind child should have maximum trouble with these terms, for they seem to refer directly to the sighted world. Nonetheless, as we will show, a congenitally blind child can acquire considerable sophistication with the sighted vocabulary.

To understand these surprising findings, we then examined the actual input circumstances of a blind learner to ascertain whether selected properties of the sentences or contexts provided by her caregivers explain the character of what she learned. The findings from this inquiry taken as a whole give little support to the view that first language attainment is explainable as a straightforward derivative of information provided in the environment of the learner. Rather, they suggest to us a learning procedure significantly modulated and constrained by the child's natural (innate) biases about the content and form of a natural language.

Before turning to our study of blind children, we want to consider the general problems learners seem to face in inducing the lexicon from observation of extralinguistic circumstances.

Three Problems for Learning from Observation

Following Locke, we have asserted that to make children understand words, people show them the thing "and then repeat to them the name that stands for it." (Of course the settings for such showing and telling usually are informal rather than overtly tutorial but this does not change the position.) Still there is a problem because of the particularities of these learning experiences as compared with the generality of what is learned. The child who has seen Fido and Rover while hearing the sound signal /dɔg/ will ultimately be able—without further language learning—to refer to Rex and Spot by producing the same sound signal. That is, the child's input consists of sound/situation pairs, but his final output is a set of form/meaning pairs, appropriate to an infinite set of novel but well-circumscribed situations. How is it that children ineluctably move from these singular experiences to general knowledge of terms, which allows their creative use? How do they project to the full set of pairings in the language—all dogs from Pekinese to Russian wolfhounds—given the small and inconclusive subset of pairings—say, Chihuahuas and poodles—provided by experience? To help understand the issues here, we now take up three problems in making good the claim that language can be learned "from" experience.

Too many encodings of experience are available

Normally circumstanced learners are exposed to objects, scenes, and events as they listen to the stream of speech. But these objects, scenes, and events are in no direct way the "meanings" that learners are seeking to pair with the language forms. They are merely what they seem to be: objects, scenes, and events. Any of them can be linguistically described in myriad ways, for language can encode a variety of descriptions of a single scene. For instance, the same creature out there is an object, a mammal, a cat, Felix. And the same event out there is the cat on the mat, the mat under the cat, and the mat and the cat on the floor. When the cat is pointed to (accompanied by the sound /kæt/), then, what is to prevent the listening-watching child from interpreting that experience (and that sound) as 'object,' 'organism,' 'furriness,' 'white,' 'cute,' 'whiskers,' 'legs'?[2]

Similarly, scenes relevant to the utterance "The cat is on the mat" are just as relevant to "The mat is under the cat" or "The cat and the mat are on the floor." How is the learner to realize that the linguistic encoding (the *particular* sentence spoken) is of one of these descriptions of the scene and not the other? The real-world context available to the learner is apposite to all of them.

The problem, in short, is that there is always as much positive evidence in the external world for one of these interpretations as for the next. If no child chooses the false solutions, the question is how they all know enough to avoid them. If some of the children do choose falsely—that is, if we settle on different internal constructions of the sense of words—the problem is how we ever manage to understand each other. Thus the general acknowledgment that context is necessary should not be confused with a proof that it is sufficient for language acquisition. That is why one can't (though many do) say the child learns language from observing the world, and let it go at that.

These problems are extremely tricky. One false conjecture about the particular sentence spoken by the adult, and an escalating series of miscalculations about the language is likely to ensue. For example, suppose the child guesses the unintended mat-under-cat interpretation while she is hearing a cat-on-mat utterance. Then she might conclude (falsely, of course) that *cat* means 'mat' and *on* means 'under.' But this simple reversal is not the only wrong direction she might take. After all, she comes equipped with no passport to tell her that the language in question is English and that therefore the subject probably comes before the verb; other languages systematically use a different ordering of thematic roles in simple sentences. Thus the learner who has made the accidentally false conjecture about the scene description (mat-under-cat) while hearing "cat on mat" may correctly conjecture that *cat* means 'cat,' but at the cost of the false conjecture that English is an object-first rather than a subject-first language—and, again, that *on* means 'under.' No wonder, in light of such problems, that the mere statement that learning relies on contextual interpretation has achieved little in the way of definite results, nor been able to explain what is learned when and under what conditions by children.[3]

False experiences

It must be true that occasionally a child is inspecting a scene while the adult is thinking and speaking of something else altogether, creating a potentially false pairing for the inductive learner. For example, a mother might say "Granny is coming for dinner" or "Time for your nap" while the child inspects a cat on the mat. What is to prevent the learner from the attempt to pair this extralinguistic experience with the sound signal /taɪmfəryərnæp/? If this problem is not qualitatively different from those mentioned just above, it certainly is an exacerbation of the real difficulties in envisaging a machinery that extracts the words and their meanings from raw confrontations with utterance/event pairs.

The problem of abstract meanings

A great many words, among them many that are easily learned by toddlers, have no direct connection with sensory-perceptual experience. Whatever the basis for learning words that refer to rabbits, waistcoats, and watchfobs, much of the lexicon traffics in concepts that overreach in abstractness what any child can be expected to induce from immediate environmental cues. Even such simple verbs as *get* or *put* require for felicitous use apprehension of a mental goal, not just an action, on the part of the speaker/listener (for discussion, see Huttenlocher, Smiley, and Charney, 1983). Even such simple nouns as *fun* and *pet*, or adjectives such as *fair* and *good*, encode descriptions not embodied in the physical substance or single material property of their extensions. In addition, some words encode highly general and often unobservable relations (*similar, brother, but*) and properties (*very, the*) or grammatical functions divorced from any experiential description (*of* or infinitival *to*). But learners evidently have little trouble in acquiring the sense of these words, which could not derive from material aspects of experience.

Constraining the Inductive Machinery

The problems just mentioned are well known. Of course they obtain only if it is assumed that the learner is openminded about the categories he is willing to form and about the observational conditions under which he is disposed to make a conjecture about word meanings. But if the learner truly is like an all-purpose general learning machine, taking each experience as an appropriate condition for forming an induction, there is no end of hypotheses, some absurd but many reasonable, it can entertain as construals of a single scene. Real language learning simply cannot look like this. Details that are required for a realistic theory include (merely!) specific descriptions of sensation, perception, and cognition which assure that humans are disposed by nature to interpret their experience as cat-experiences in preference to cat-whiskers, to undetached cat-parts, or to adventitious properties of objects and events. Such a theory is not provided by those who have maintained that there is no mystery in learning language, arguing that the feat is accomplished solely by the learner's "extralinguistic context" or "real-world experience." For the theory of observation-based learning, though surely true at least in part, is vacuous unless it specifies two components: It must elucidate the vocabulary in which experience is couched, and it must specify an inductive machinery that is somehow sensitive to the impoverishment and degeneracy of the information it receives. We now discuss some directions that such inquiries have taken.

Describing and limiting the categories of experience

So far we have taken the view that there is no limit on the categories a young learner might be willing to form on the basis of an experience with the real world. And we have tried to show that one makes little progress so long as one remains uncommitted about the essence and scope of these categories. But certainly attempts, formal and informal, have been made to respond to this inadequacy. A well-articulated approach to an exhaustive and plausible description came from the British empiricists' sensationist approach to the primary categorization of experience (though to be sure this account has foundered on data). This position (Locke, 1690; Berkeley, 1709; Hume, 1758) asserts that there is an atomic kind of experience to which the mind reacts immediately. Exposure to such experience triggers formation of the relevant concept, and then the concept is tied to its lexical encoding by association. For example, it is seeing a red patch while hearing "red" that constitutes both the condition for learning *red* and the content of that learning.

Accepting this view, the problem remains to describe the acquisition of even concrete terms that do not have a simple sensory account. For example, the word *lemon* would appear to encode at least the three categories 'yellow,' 'round,' and 'sour.' Locke proposed an answer to this problem. In his view, all categories not in the primary basis, including *lemon,* were to be built up by associative combinations of the primary ones when they co-occur in experience. Schematically, for example, the complex lexical category *lemon* is constructed given that one observes roundness, sourness, and yellowness simultaneously and, at the same time, hears the utterance "lemon."

A major implausibility in this position from most modern perspectives is the restriction of primary experience to sensory categories such as 'red' or 'A-flat' or 'sour.' Evidence that even so simple a word as *lemon* can be described as a combination of such sensory categories has simply not been forthcoming, and not for want of some hundreds of years of trying (for discussion, see Fodor, 1981, ch. 10; Armstrong, Gleitman, and Gleitman, 1983). For instance, one could inject sugar into the lemon, paint it red, and squash it, and it would still be a lemon for all its deformations—a problem that in fact Locke discussed quite revealingly (Book 3.VI.4) but did not resolve. These difficulties by themselves, however, do not greatly damage the essence of this kind of position on word learning. There is no *necessary* connection between empiricist thought and the sensory analysis of primary experience unless, like Locke, the empiricist in question is a sensationist.

Most modern empiricists countenance higher-level primary perceptual categories that humans are assumed to share (see E. Clark, 1973, who suggests that young children's word use is explainable in these terms). On some views (J. J. Gibson, 1979; E. J. Gibson and Walker, 1984, and for an adaptation to children's language learning, Nelson, 1974), the categories yielded up immediately by perception are sufficient for extracting high-level functional interpretations (*chair* might be learnable owing to an innate ability to observe the world immediately in terms of sit-upon-able-ness). Eleanor Rosch and her collaborators (1978; Rosch, Mervis, Gray, Johnson, and Boyes-Braem, 1976) have presented evidence supporting the idea that there are certain middle level or "basic" categories (more abstract than such categories as 'yellow' or 'four-legged' but less abstract than such categories as 'animal' or 'furniture') which humans are biased to construct (see Diamond, 1966, and Berlin, Breedlove, and Raven, 1974, who have demonstrated striking cross-cultural agreement in such basic categorizations of simple concrete nouns; and Mervis and Pani, 1980, Mervis and Crisafi, 1978, for adaptation to the language-learning situation).[4] In addition, many contributors to the language-learning literature have adopted the assumption that there is an *a priori* set of semantic-relational categories (cases, or thematic roles, to use the terminology preferred by some linguists), more closely tied to language itself, which learners bring to the task of discovering their native tongue (this assumption can be recognized in investigators as disparate in viewpoint as Brown, 1973; Braine and Hardy, 1982; Gleitman and Wanner, 1982, 1984; Bates and MacWhinney, 1982; and Pinker, 1984).

In sum, recent investigators differ from their predecessors by expanding the essence and number of primary categories. Postulation of these higher-level categories provides renewed vigor and plausibility to the empiricist approach to language learning. At least we are no longer confronted with the requirement, evidently impossible to meet, to build dogs and lemons from sensory impressions alone.

But this change in the postulated inductive basis raises problems of its own. Discovery of the set of atomic categories—circumscribed well enough on the British empiricist position—now becomes a wide-open topic whose dimensions are not easy to foresee. The immediate consequence for a plausible learning theory is not altogether encouraging: The greater the number of categories in terms of which the learner can react to the same scene or event, the more difficult it must become for him to select exactly which of these is encoded by a particular word or expression he then hears. As elsewhere in language studies (cf. Chomsky, 1975), the new challenge set by the expansion of the categorial base has provoked a search for constraints or at least biases in the learner as to plausible ways that the lexicon carves the real world. We shall return to discussion of the literature on this topic in Chapter 9, after we have documented the lexical inductions of blind individuals.

Specifying the inductive learning machinery

A comparable liberalization of strategies for manipulating the data provided by external experience characterizes most modern approaches to the problem of word learning. Simple association is no longer the only mechanism countenanced. Locke himself foreshadowed the view that, to explain complex lexical categories, the mind must be capable of more than the passive intake of external experience together with the automatic formation of associations among the co-occurring experiences. Thus he introduced a monumental hedge into the position that learning is from the outside in by postulating a "reflective" capacity as part of the human equipment: The mind, contemplating its own structure and content, constructs "complex ideas." We now mention in brief some hypotheses about the inductive machinery for organizing experience that have been offered in the interest of taming induction to make it a bit more realistic.

Distributional analysis

A venerable idea for understanding both language and its learning is to analyze the (relative) distributional patterns in which particular morphemes occur within the string of morphemes that comprises an utterance (Bloomfield, 1933; Harris, 1951). This kind of analysis was first proposed as a means of uncovering distinctive privileges of occurrence for morphemes that are members of the same form class. Extraction of these patterns thus could constitute a discovery procedure for those form classes. Maratsos and Chalkley (1980) and Maratsos (1982) have investigated such form/form patterns in detail and argue quite persuasively that children might discover from them, e.g., which morphemes are the nouns and which are the verbs in the utterances they hear. For instance, the verbs might be just those morphemes that occur after *will* and *can* and before *-ed*.

However, insofar as the sentence is conceived simply as a linear string of morphemes, it turns out to be very difficult to render such a procedure practical. For example, some of the *-ed*'s do not come after verbs at all. While *-ed* follows a verb in *hotfooted* or *hightailed*, it follows an adjective in *lightfingered* and *bobtailed*; thus appearance before *-ed* is not a secure criterion for assigning verb status to a morpheme. Gleitman and Wanner (1982; 1984) have discussed the problems with this kind of inductive machinery and propose that a phrase-structural description of the input utterance might provide a format within which a distributional scheme such as Maratsos' might be more likely to succeed (see Chapter 7 for further discussion). However, the *hightailed/bobtailed* example will suffice here to suggest that any such scheme must involve storage of a very large number of sentences either in an unanalyzed form or at best analyzed only very provisionally.

Despite the apparent burden on memory and computation such schemes would seem to necessitate, there certainly is no knockdown logical argument against them. Moreover, they seem especially attractive when they are assumed to take form/meaning pairings as input (Wexler and Culicover, 1980) rather than just form/form pairings (Bloomfield or Maratsos). Some problems of word learning might then be approachable. The assumption would be that the learner has a large memory store in his head for squirreling away situation/utterance pairs. Some of these will be correct (the situation cat-on-mat paired with the utterance "The cat is on the mat"), and of course some will be incorrect (cat-on-mat paired with "The mat is under the cat"). But the learner need not choose precipitately between these provisional pairings. Perhaps he can hold *cat/mat* choices and syntactic format choices in abeyance until he has enough data to manipulate comparatively: Eventually there will occur cat-scenes without mats, mat-scenes without cats, naps without cats, and the like, in his environment. These dissociating sound/event circumstances possibly can be exploited to resolve the problems of acquiring the meanings of words.

A learner operating in this way would be wary of making *any* inductive generalization based on a single or a very small number of received situation/utterance pairs. Rather he would somehow store the pairs in his head until he had enough of them to consider against each other. Once the input corpus is large, he would have a basis for the claim that "Time for your nap" was an utterance that was not—over the data base as a whole—in any strong way contingent on whether there were cats or for that matter any objects at all in view.

The trouble is that when we consider such schemes in detail, they again seem to place an unreasonable memorial and computational burden on the learning machinery. The learner who hears "the cat on the mat" paired with the situation of cat-on-mat must hang onto the pair, unanalyzed, waiting for lucky circumstance to offer "the rat is on the mat." Now holding mats constant, the learner perhaps is in a position to recognize that the cats and the rats are the animals, not the carpets. But how long must he wait, for each such unanalyzed pair, before the crucial dissociating second or third or hundredth pair comes along? But matters are even worse than this. Luck in the input conditions is also needed lest he hear "the mat is on the floor" the next time he sees a cat on the mat.

All in all, making good on a distributional scheme for establishing the form/meaning pairings seems to require a formidable retention of unanalyzed material or else many contingent inductions that have to be revised under the pressure of continuously arriving new pairings. Even if the learner has the sophisticated storage and manipulative capacities required, the predictions from this kind of machinery do not seem to square with the known findings in the language-learning literature. First, we ought to expect a large number of errors to be made by young children—sometimes they should call cats "mat" depending on the luck of the draw. But this phenomenon is rare to the point of invisibility. The only frequent errors observed in meaning assignments are those that have to do with the generality of a category (*ball* might be used for all round things, including faces and the moon), and even these mistakes are largely restricted to the very earliest stages of acquisition (during appearance of the first seventy-five words early in the second year of life, Rescorla, 1980).

Second, again taking into account the luck of the draw, there ought to be great disparities in the early vocabularies of youngsters, but instead their early vocabularies are strikingly alike over quite different exposure conditions (Nelson, 1973; Feldman, Goldin-Meadow, and Gleitman, 1978; and see Chapter 2 for evidence from blind learners). More generally, if the inductive schema we are considering is the right one, we ought to predict large differences in the rate of language learning by various youngsters in various language communities, raised under differing child-rearing practices with the differences in utterances heard that this implies (for instance, the Kaluli hardly speak to their young children for the first few years of life, considering them not yet human, while middle-class American mothers seem to take the reverse position, Schieffelin, 1982). But the language-acquisition literature reveals a striking uniformity across individuals, languages, and cultures in the growth of a first language during the first five years of life. These difficulties, while they do not logically dispose of the distributional proposal, certainly provide some impetus for seeking at least auxiliary apparatus in the young learner.

Further inductive principles

Even if we have just shown the difficulty of a particular inductive machinery, there surely are many other such schemes, containing certain corrective properties, that we have not addressed. But our intention was simply to give a first hint about the scope of the problem faced by a relatively naked inductive device that sets out to acquire meanings from situation/utterance pairs. Modern investigators in both psychology and philosophy have moved in a rather different direction. They have given significant attention to the development of learning principles and strategies more complex and at the same time more constrained than simple association or raw distributional analysis. Often these are formal attempts to describe concepts that will be difficult to attain from experience, not because of a restriction on the categories of experience themselves, but because of restrictions on how inductive logics are to work given the phenomena they are to explain. Examples are Goodman's (1966) calculus for extensional simplicity, Sommers' (1959) description of "predicability trees," and Osherson's (1978) adaptation of Fitch logic to describe natural connectives. Basically, the point of this enterprise is to explain the content and logic of concepts that are acquired easily as opposed to those that experience may make available and yet are hard to acquire, thus making induction possible by constraining its operation.

Adaptation of these and related ideas within empirical studies of word and concept learning can be found in the recent literature (for an excellent discussion, see Osherson, 1978). For example, Bever and Rosenbaum (1970) and Keil (1979) propose a description of the organization among the lexical entries that is strictly hierarchical. Given this constraint, no new word, regardless of the contexts in which it is heard, could encode the idea 'either some living thing or some event' for *living thing* and *event* occupy established, distinct, higher nodes in a semantic hierarchy into which this proposed new item must fit. To take a specific example, a word meaning 'your bed and when you sleep' might be outlawed, thus reining in the interpretation of *time* in "Time for your nap" (see also Markman and Hutchinson, 1984). Billman (1983) has proposed that the inductive procedure becomes more refined over time and experience. It examines those features that have so far been implicated in the correct inductions about words, and highlights these—dampening others—as probably the material ones for yet further inductions. Shipley and Kuhn (1983) make a related claim in their theory of "equally detailed alternatives." Their supposition is that those properties that have served to construct one lexical entry (e.g., a specification of color, size, habitat, and gait for robins) will suggest to the learner that the next bird must be specified on the same dimensions.

All these suggestions have to do with the format for the child's induction of lexical entries and the manipulations that can be performed within the constraints imposed by the formats. All of them thus make induction from experience easier by assigning more structure and processing power to the child learner than was envisaged by, say, John Locke. Many of these proposals also incorporate the idea that inductive learning changes over the course of development as a consequence of progress already made. For example, Carey (forthcoming) has urged that the learning child constructs intuitive theories, e.g., a primitive physics, biology, and psychology, whose internal organization must be respected by new lexical items. Keil and Batterman (1984) have some evidence which suggests that category construction shifts from prototypical structures early in life to close to definitional ones later on (but see Landau, 1982a, for an alternative view). Kemler (1983) has shown that the young child is inclined toward 'holistic' categorizations of experience, but that these become dimensionalized and analytic as cognitive growth proceeds. In general, many investigators have proposed that the construction of categories changes with development, based on growing knowledge of language and its structure (Markman and Huchinson, 1984; Shipley, Kuhn, and Madden, 1983), knowledge acquisition (Chi, 1978; Carey, forthcoming), and prior lexical acquisitions (Shipley and Kuhn, 1983; Billman, 1983).

In sum, the general problem of learning a first language is materially altered depending on the machinery granted for forming and organizing the categories of experience. The proposals both for enriching and for constraining the categories, and the combinatorial machinery that binds them, are attempts to respond to the fact that induction unrestrained in operating principles and unrefined in the categories entertained is almost surely too weak to account for the real facts of lexical learning: acquiring about the same set of words, with about the same meanings, within about the same time period, under widely varying exposure conditions.

Special Problems of the Blind Learner

Blind children seem to approach the task of language learning deprived of many opportunities to observe the world that language is describing. Though they can explore objects haptically, sighted children can explore them both haptically and visually. Even on the presumption that manual exploration can straightforwardly substitute for visual exploration, the practical facts both about conversational interactions and about stimulus objects often place the blind child at a disadvantage for testing and confirming conjectures about word meaning. For example, sometimes the blind learner is too far away to experience the rabbit or cup or doll that is under discussion. For certain objects, the differences in the experiences available to blind and sighted child are qualitative and severe. The colors of rabbits are visible only—in principle. Shapes of certain things (those too large, distant, or gossamer to explore by hand, such as mountains, birds, and fog) are visible only—in practice.

To put some initial perspective to our investigations of blind

learners, we now review what is currently known about their initial competencies and early progress. These, we believe, make a
prima facie case that the environment of blind learners is restricted
and deficient in ways that might be expected to bear on lexical
concept attainment. Thus they provide a test case for how learning can proceed when the circumstances of observation are dramatically changed.

Exploratory capacities of the young blind child

Vision clearly is not the only window to the world. Would anyone
doubt, for example, that blind and sighted infants should be completely on a par in the discrimination and recognition of odors
and tastes? It has even been suggested that the blind may excel in
such nonvisual discriminations, since these would be bound to be
exercised more than they are for the sighted (Jones, 1972; see
Warren, 1977, for further examples). However, neither taste nor
odor seems to provide much information for learning about the
objects, properties, and events that form the underlying conceptual layer supporting language learning. Potentially more important are the haptic and aural senses. As for the latter, it is simply a
fact that neither concepts nor the words that label them—a few
onomatopoetic instances such as *cuckoo* and *bobwhite* excepted—
are discoverable directly from auditory information (the sound
/tut-tut/ provides inferential evidence that a train may be nearby,
but *toot-toot* doesn't mean 'train,' at least not for long). By elimina-
tion, then, argument about whether a blind child is likely to learn
language unexceptionally has usually come down to the question
of whether the haptic system can adequately substitute for the
visual system in constructing a spatial world populated by objects,
properties, and events.

   The literature on tactile-haptic perception informs us that, at
least for older children, adults, and other species, one can be fairly
optimistic about the prospects for constructing a spatial world
similar to that of sighted people from the hands, limbs, and body
moving through space (Gordon, 1978; Schiff and Foulke, 1982).
Spatial properties such as the position of one's body and the
weight, size, and texture of objects can be detected without vision
(see Ruff, 1984, who examined aspects of this issue with sighted
infants). Moreover, such sophisticated symbolic representations
as drawings can be understood by the blind (Kennedy, 1978).
Older blind children and adults can also understand and use tactile maps to guide locomotion without the use of vision (Leonard

and Newman, 1967; Armstrong, 1978; Berla, 1982; and for a demonstration with a young blind child, Landau, 1984a).

But even if spatial learning can take place in the absence of vision, this does not suggest that the hand is really *equivalent* to the eye, especially in early development. The question is if and when manual exploration becomes a fully adequate substitute for visual search and inspection. The picture here is complex. In sighted children, systematic visual exploration seems to precede haptic exploration developmentally (Warren, 1982, and Berla, 1982, for reviews). Visual exploration begins in early infancy (Haith, 1980). Sighted infants display at least the rudiments of visually guided reaching as newborns (Hofsten, 1982). By four months, they show coordination between vision and audition (Spelke, 1979) and, somewhat later, between vision and manual/oral haptic exploration (Gottfried, Rose, and Bridger, 1977; Rose, Gottfried, and Bridger, 1981).

In contrast, blind infants are reputed to be passive, using their hands only in the service of bringing things to the mouth, and engaging in active manual exploration relatively late in development. Some information comes from Fraiberg (1977), who conducted a longitudinal study of ten congenitally blind children. She showed that they were much more likely than sighted infants to be delayed in self-initiated motor behaviors (e.g., walking and crawling, though not sitting and standing). Further, she showed that blind infants did not reach toward a sounding object until about eleven months—six months later than sighted infants are typically found to reach toward a seen object.[5]

To understand this finding, it is essential to replicate it with sighted infants. The relevant studies are from Freedman, Fox-Kolenda, Margileth, and Miller (1969). They found that sighted infants performed exactly as the blind infants did, reaching toward objects based on sound cues alone only much later than they would reach toward objects based on visual cues. Similarly, Bigelow (1983, 1984) has shown that sound is a late elicitor of object search in infancy. These findings do not suggest that blind children have a necessary or long-lasting deficit in object representation. Rather they show that sound is a later elicitor of reaching behavior for any infant—blind or sighted—than is vision. Vision provides "information that one should reach toward" (or "affords" that information, in Gibson's terms) before sound gives that information during the development of the infant. The young blind child is thus necessarily delayed in his exploration of the spatial world beyond his body. This probabilistically reduces the chances that he is in (manual) contact with an object when it is being talked about, compared to the chances that a sighted child is in (either or both) manual or visual contact with an object when it is being talked about.

Once blind children do begin to explore the world around them, what can one predict for their subsequent development of knowledge of objects, properties, and events in the world and their linguistic encodings? Again the situation is complex, for haptic exploration is only a partial substitute for vision in providing information for the identification of objects. Putting the problem generally, in order to construct a spatial array one needs to explore its parts and to plot them in memory relative to each other and to some appropriate reference system. The question is whether blind children can construct such a coherent array from the partial and sequential information afforded through touch.

Our own studies suggest that a blind two-year-old is capable of making spatial inferences in certain circumstances. She can construct knowledge of a large spatial array after successive walks along parts of that array (Landau, H. Gleitman, and Spelke, 1981; Landau, Spelke, and H. Gleitman, 1984). These findings demonstrate that vision is not required for the construction and manipulation of spatial arrays from successive exposures to their parts. They lend support to observations made by others on the surprising capacities of young blind children to find their way about familiar environments (Norris, Spaulding, and Brodie, 1957; Adelson, 1983) and on the later competencies of the blind in performing a variety of spatial tasks (Jones, 1975).

However, other studies suggest that the blind child up to the age of about four has some remaining problems in organizing experience. At least until then, shape recognition by certain kinds of tactile exploration is not achieved with any facility, by either blind or sighted children. Indeed, it has been suggested that only later in development can haptic exploration be used as a ready substitute for visual search (Piaget and Inhelder, 1948/67; Zaporzhets, 1965; Abravanel, 1968, 1970). Several causal factors have been suggested for why it might be difficult to identify shapes by hand early in life. For one thing, there may be poorer retention of tactile than visual information under certain circumstances (Rose, Blank, and Bridger, 1972; Millar, 1974; Sullivan and Turvey, 1972). Moreover, some kinds of haptic exploration seem to lead naturally to the construction of textural and density dimensions rather than dimensions relevant to shape. For instance, Millar (1978) showed that blind children tend to group braille characters according to their similarities in the density of dots rather than according to the overall shapes of the dot designs (for related findings, see Abravanel, 1970; Lederman, 1978). Perhaps most important, even neonates have been shown to explore arrays visually in terms of a systematic strategy in which a spontaneous reference system is recruited; in contrast, some kinds of early haptic explorations tend to be nonsystematic (Millar, 1978). Note that this finding does not contradict the spatial learning work of Landau et al. with blind children. In our experiments, an obvious—though by no means "given"—reference system was provided for the child by always aligning her at the origin during exposure to the array.

Summarizing, there is evidence that vision is not a requirement for spatial construction under all circumstances. Still the blind child seems to be at a disadvantage at least up to about age four in constructing object shapes when there is no obvious reference system available. These difficulties diminish in later childhood. Thus though some difficulties may be expected owing to the developmental timing and the internal functions readily computed in nonvisual modalities, haptic exploration would seem eventually to provide a solid basis for interacting with the world that language encodes. Though learning might be late and even deviant in subtle ways, we are not wholly at a loss in explaining that—to the extent language *is* learned from experience—blind learners have a means for gaining that experience.

Interactions between the blind child and her sighted caregivers

But there is another potential obstacle for blind children: They must learn by interaction with sighted caregivers whose experiences differ from their own. It is this fact that we believe poses the most devastating challenge to the blind learner. The sighted mother and child evolve naturally into a pointing, gesturing, mutually indicating pair who can capitalize on the spatial properties of vision (Bruner, 1974–75). By the age of eight months, the sighted child can follow his mother's pointing gesture and infer by straightforward triangulation what her object of attention is. By age twelve months the child can use the same devices to draw adults' attention (Collis, 1977; Schaffer, 1977; Butterworth, 1983). As Bruner suggested, language learning would certainly seem to be aided to the extent that tutor and learner can be sure they are attending to and referring to the same things, scenes, and events. Masur (1982) found that mothers are inclined to provide object names when children point. And children, in their turn, produce object names when mothers point. Reasonably enough, Masur concludes that these pointing activities lead to vocabulary learning (see also Ninio and Bruner, 1978; Ninio, 1980).

Is there a haptic or aural equivalent for these co-attentive visual devices, used by blind children and their parents? Certainly the mother and child can together or sequentially hold the same object, and the blind child can explore it by his own haptic means if the object is a small one. Even for a large object, he can explore and record certain properties such as texture or sound. Mother and blind learner can jointly name objects that each is exploring by these differing means. Urwin (1983) has shown that mothers and their blind children do use these alternate strategies for focussing their joint attention. What is unclear is whether these special strategies work as well as the pointing and mutual gesturing of sighted people are said to do. Certain details of blind toddlers' language use suggest struggles in trying to encode the ambiant world of things and events. Sometimes their utterances seem incomprehensible and irrelevant to sighted listeners; they initiate comments and other verbal interactions much more rarely than sighted children of the same age; and their sentences often refer to their own bodily state rather than to the world outside the body (Burlingham, 1964; Urwin, 1983). All this suggests that there are continuing practical difficulties in encoding the world of objects and events by blind children, and in coordinating these encodings with linguistic formatives (the words and phrases of the language being learned).

Pragmatic consequences of exploratory differences: The Miss Piggy Teapot Problem

To understand the problems a blind learner faces in practice, it may be helpful to consider a specific incident. We had told a blind three-year-old, Kelli, about a Miss Piggy Teapot, which Kelli then demanded to examine (actually she asked "to see it," but *that* runs well ahead of our story). The top of the teapot consisted of Miss Piggy's hat, complete with three-dimensional glass cherries as adornments, and her head. The teapot bottom represented all of Miss Piggy, head excepted. Feeling her way along this object, Kelli identified two of the cherries in the teapot top as Miss Piggy's eyes, and the bottom margin of the teapot top (the bottom of the head) as Miss Piggy's mouth. Well, why not? Nothing bizarre about these conjectures. They just happen to be wrong. It is the difficulties of conducting the unsystematic haptic search and the fact that Miss Piggy's parts are *really* disambiguated by paint colors in this object that account for Kelli's problem in arriving at the veridical solution.

These practicalities continually plague young blind children in handling the pragmatics of everyday conversation, for they often cannot figure out what is occurring in the ongoing social event. Imagine the difficulty of taking part in a conversation in which all the participants—yourself excepted—are present together, while you are connected to them only by telephone. One common result for blind children, including those we studied, is lateness in disentangling the personal pronouns. A related finding is that sometimes blind children (again, including our own subjects) engage in private speech play, apparently unrelated to ongoing events, which is hard for sighted adults to understand and is often interpreted as autistic (for discussion, see Fraiberg, 1977).

The question, then, is not whether the blind child's experience differs from that of the sighted learner. Of course it does. As just stated, they *are* often confused about events taking place around them, and they *do* sometimes behave in asocial and conversationally incompetent ways that border on the bizarre. Thus the idea that blind children suffer a deprivation of experience is not just theoretically possible; it is practically demonstrable. Moreover, these deprivations affect the conversational competencies of the blind at least up to the third birthday.

The Blind Experience and Language Learning

We might now seem to have answered the question with which we began: The blind do suffer a deprivation of experience, and that deprivation is manifest in their early understanding of the world around them and of conversations. But this was not really our question. The question we hope to engage is how learners acquire the relations between lexical forms and their meanings. Though we have just shown that the blind two-year-old has difficulties in figuring out what is going on and therefore in conversing competently, this does not necessarily mean that she therefore is unable to learn the meanings of words and sentences. This is an empirical question that cannot be answered simply by alluding to the real-life difficulties that a blind learner faces.

Suppose—as we will document—that the blind child really can acquire the meanings of words and sentences. And suppose—as we just described—that he or she must do so in the presence of a somewhat deficient understanding of real-world events and attendant conversational niceties. If both suppositions are correct, then the relations between "experiencing what is going on" and "acquiring the English language" must be more dissociable than some have supposed.

Restating, our question is whether the demonstrable differences between the blind and the sighted in their early opportunities to observe the here-and-now are relevant and sufficiently pervasive that they inevitably predict an abnormal course for language learning in the blind population. Such investigators as Bloom (1983) have asserted as a matter of theoretical principle that a blind child must be deficient in *language*, that even though blind children come to say words and sentences, they have "disordered language," "speech that is disjunctive in its meaning," because they are "deprived of normal input from the context."

This is not true, as we shall show. After a possible mild delay in onset and transient confusions with personal pronouns, blind children go on to acquire language that in form and content, and in application to the real world of things, events, and scenes, is altogether unexceptional. In fact, the rate of this learning is not even particularly slow. Now it follows either that the role of context in language acquisition has been overestimated, or that context must be analyzed in a new way, a way that allows us to say that the blind child's situation is hardly disadvantaged at all.

In later discussion (Chapters 7 and 9), we will invoke both of these possibilities to explain the linguistic success of the blind. We will suggest that human learners' specific dispositions concerning the form and contents of a natural language allow them to override many otherwise expectable effects of situational oddities and deficiencies. Moreover, higher-order analyses of context, which transcend the specific differences in information afforded by the individual senses, place the child in a position to learn through the ambient environment. Where the eye is missing, the hand may provide adequate input to a learning device that maps onto converging central representations.

Finally, a point often missed is that part of the child's experiential context is linguistic. Very early in the learning process, the systematicity of the language code becomes available to the learner at least in its rudiments. To the extent that the language system is organized in semantically relevant ways, it serves as an important bootstrap into ever more subtle discoveries about the linguistic means for communication. In short, a critical contextual cue to language learning is language itself.

To reiterate our general purpose: We accept as self-evident that all children learn language based on speech and contextual information which underdetermines the system that generates it. Blind learners serve to dramatize the reality of this problem, for they suffer obvious experiential deprivations. This is why, given our interest in understanding the normal induction of language, we have studied the blind child.

2 / The Development of Speech in Blind Children

B oth for syntax and for word learning, the view that experience is necessary and sufficient predicts late learning and long-term deficits for the blind. Accordingly, we studied vocabulary and syntactic development in blind youngsters using standard measures by which they could be compared to sighted children of the same ages. As will be shown, blind children begin to speak rather late, though within the normal range; thereafter the prognosis for normal speech development in otherwise intact blind youngsters is very good indeed. By the third birthday, they are virtually indistinguishable from their sighted peers.

A few large-scale studies of this population already exist. These serve to establish norms for two milestones in language attainment: language onset (measured as a vocabulary of two words) and syntax onset (measured as the first appearance of two-word sentences). But more detail than this is required to answer the question of whether the blind develop normal speech within the usual time periods. To fill the gap, we conducted detailed and repeated interviews and measurements of our subjects. The scope of this testing limited the number of children we could realistically investigate to three individuals whose families were willing to allow us to interview the children in many sessions, extending over two to four years. This small sample size is the norm in longitudinal studies of spontaneous speech development, which have substituted many measurements of a few individuals for a few measurements of many (and such studies, e.g. Brown, 1973, Bloom, Lightbown, and Hood, 1975, have stood up remarkably well in replications with further subjects, learning various languages).

The Blind Subjects

Kelli

Kelli is the firstborn of two children, with a sighted sister twelve months younger. Kelli was the survivor of a pair of twins born approximately three months prematurely. She was very small (weight 940 grams at birth) and ill and was immediately placed in an isolette. The oxygen-rich environment of the isolette resulted in a condition called retrolental fibroplasia (RLF), which blinded her (grade-4 RLF in the left eye and grade-5 RLF in the right eye). She was diagnosed as totally blind, though recent tests suggest she may have some sensitivity to light in one eye (enough to tell bright light from darkness, but not enough to detect shadows or shapes). Kelli remained in the hospital for six months, when she was discharged weighing approximately 6 pounds with a developmental status of newborn. Because Kelli's blindness was caused by RLF, a condition often associated also with some kinds of brain damage, we had her assessed neurologically and behaviorally during the period of observation; no other defect in function was found or suspected.

We first observed Kelli at the age of 21 months (18 months, correcting for prematurity; henceforth, we present chronological age only). At that time, it was clear that she was delayed in her motor development relative to sighted norms, as is common among blind children (Fraiberg, 1977) and is also common among premature children, even sighted ones (Gleitman and Landau, forthcoming). At the time of our first observation, Kelli was neither standing nor walking independently. She walked with support at 22 months, stood independently at 24 months, and walked independently at 26 months. While this is a considerable deviation from sighted norms, it falls within the range for congenitally blind children (Fraiberg, 1977). Socially, Kelli seemed happy, active, and cooperative.

We observed Kelli an average of every three weeks from the first observation at 21 months through her fifth birthday. The spontaneous speech samples were collected from her first words at 23 months through her complex sentences at 42 months.

Carlo

Carlo is the secondborn of three children, with one sighted sister eight years older and another two and a half years younger. Carlo was born approximately two and one half months prematurely, weighing 1500 grams. Aside from the more common distresses of prematurity, he was not particularly ill and remained in the hospital isolette for only six weeks. During that time, like Kelli, he became a victim of RLF. He was left with grade-3 RLF in one eye and grade-4 RLF in the other. This means he was considered to have probable light perception in the better eye. There are clear behavioral indications that he does have some ability to tell light from dark and can even detect shadows and gross shapes. For instance, as an infant and toddler he habitually dug at the better eye, possibly to receive more light stimulation; he amused himself by passing objects including his own hand in front of the better eye; he anticipated objects in his path, reaching out to touch them before actually making contact. In light of these capacities, one might wonder why we included Carlo in the sample. The answer is that he had an extreme enough visual handicap for our investigative purposes. He displayed significant "blindisms," such as rocking, digging at the eye, exploring objects by mouth in the early years of life, showing preference for noise-making objects, being late in acquiring first words, and showing extensive verbal imitation and incorrect referential use of pronouns (for comparison with other blind youngsters, see Fraiberg, 1977).

Despite Carlo's visual handicap, his gross motor development closely approximated sighted norms. At our first observation at 13 months he was standing independently. He walked with support at 14 months and walked independently at 17 months. Speech samples were collected from his first words at 26 months through complex syntax at 42 months. Speech samples were collected about every month after the onset of language and about every two months once he started combining words within sentences. Socially, Carlo fell squarely in the normal behavioral range. He was assessed periodically for neurological and behavioral damage, and no defects were found.

Angie

Angie is the firstborn of two children, with a sighted sister two years younger. Angie was the product of a normal full-term birth, but was found to have a congenital visual defect causing blindness. She has been diagnosed as having deficient optic nerve growth and macular development and has no light perception in her left eye, with some probable light perception in her right eye.

Angie was first observed when she was 29 months old and already a fluent speaker, ahead of the norms for sighted children of the same age. Her mother reported that all developmental milestones had occurred on a normal time course. She walked independently at 12 months, said her first words before 12 months, and combined words by 18 months, by maternal report. Our own subsequent observations confirmed this precocity in language learning during its later stages. Since Angie was fairly well advanced at our first observation, we visited her only once every few months (from 29 months to 42 months) to track further development. Like Kelli and Carlo, Angie is an active and friendly child. She was assessed periodically for neurological and behavioral damage and no defects were found.

Summary of the Subjects

All three children were diagnosed as clinically blind and free of other neurological defects. Kelli, the child we investigated in greatest detail (in spatial as well as language studies, see Landau et al., 1981; 1984), had no light perception and only possible light sensitivity in one eye. The minimal light perception of Carlo and Angie did not allow them to explore their ambiant worlds through vision. At best, it was sufficient to help them avoid obstacles and to receive undifferentiated light stimulation.

Perhaps the best indication that these subjects were representative of the blind population was their language development itself. The early language progress of Kelli and Carlo was characteristic of that of the premature blind population as a whole, as shown in independent normative studies we will cite again later (Norris et al., 1957). The child with the most visual capacity of the three (Carlo) was the slowest of the three in language development. The child with the least visual capacity of the three (Kelli) fell between the other two in rate of language development. The third subject (Angie) fell between the other two in the visual deficit and was linguistically precocious at each point in observation (but note again that we have only maternal reports for her until age 29 months).

All three children were of middle-class background, and each was in the normal range of general cognitive, motor, and perceptual development, as measured by the Bayley Scales of Infant Development and the Stanford-Binet Tests of Intelligence.

The Onset of Speech

If language learning is dependent on extralinguistic experience, and if blind children are not in a position to get that experience very satisfactorily, our first expectation should be that learning

begins late for the blind. Indeed, some evidence in the literature
suggests that the onset of speech is relatively late for blind children (see Warren, 1977, for review). Particularly, Norris et al.
(1957) have data from eighty-six neurologically intact blind children. They do not report mean onset times for their population
(measured as two vocabulary items) but instead present the findings as a range: More than 25 percent of these youngsters had two
words at age 15 months, more than 50 percent achieved this
learning in the period from 18 to 21 months, and more than 75
percent achieved this level by 24 months. This is roughly eight
months later than onset time for sighted full-term normals, as assessed by Lenneberg's norms (1967) and by those of the Bayley
Infant Intelligence Scale. However, there is a good deal of variability in language onset for sighted normal children. The Bayley
age range for onset varies from 10 to 23 months, and about 75
percent of the Norris et al. subjects do fall within this range.

The same authors also have data on the onset of syntax (two-
word utterances). More than 25 percent of their blind subjects
achieved this level by 24 months, more than 50 percent by 27
months, and more than 75 percent by 30 months. This again
places the blind children as a group about eight months behind
Lenneberg's norms for sighted individuals. Our own two subjects
who were observed at this early point, Kelli and Carlo, said their
first words at 23 (20, correcting for prematurity) and 26 (23)
months, thus falling in the bottom quartile of the Norris et al.
range, i.e. about twelve months below Lenneberg's median figures
for sighted full-term children.

The studies just cited are not altogether definitive because there
are a number of other factors correlated with blindness that may
contribute to late onset. Among these is prematurity. Eighty-five
percent of the Norris et al. subjects were premature births (with
RLF). We have data from forty sighted children varying in gestation period (Gleitman and Landau, forthcoming) suggesting a
delay in language onset due to prematurity itself. For example,
onset of syntax for three of five sighted subjects in this sample
who had a 24–28 week gestation period (controls for Kelli and
Carlo) occurred at about 24 months, later than mean onset time
for the sighted full-term population but earlier than the Norris et
al. mean for blind children (see Figure 2.4 of this chapter). In
comparison, Kelli produced her first two-word sentences at 29
months (26, corrected for prematurity) and Carlo produced his
somewhere between 28 and 30 (25 and 27) months. Angie, who
was a full-term birth, apparently was precocious from the begin-

ning compared to normal sighted individuals, but again early data from her are from maternal report only.

Thus prematurity seems to account for a portion of blind children's delay, but by no means all of it. We cannot be sure whether other neurological and physiological correlates account for the delay, but note that both the Norris et al. and our own population were screened for gross neurological defects. Environmental factors, much harder to evaluate, seem unsatisfactory. For example, it is possible that time spent in an isolette, deprived of exposure to speech, might set the learning clock back. Again, though, our two premature subjects differed in the time spent in this apparatus but had roughly equal delays. Moreover, Carlo has a sighted sister, also born three months prematurely and hospitalized in an isolette for about the same time as Carlo. She began to speak at 12 months.

While the evidence is somewhat confusing, then, the best guess is that relatively late onset of speech is characteristic for blind children, though not all blind subjects fall below the median onset time for normals and most blind individuals do fall within the normal range.

Can a theory of language learning that stresses the role of experience account for this delay? The findings discussed in Chapter 1, concerning the development of haptic exploratory skills, suggest that it can. As will be demonstrated later, blind children can count on their haptic capacities to give them information about the world that language encodes. But the haptic skills do not seem to have the requisite precision in the same prespeech period (roughly the first year of life) during which, presumably, sighted children are beginning to learn about the world and how language describes it. Thus even if haptic exploration can substitute for visual exploration in providing the contextual support for language learning, initial delay for a blind learner is predicted by this biologically imposed constraint on the opportunity to experience the world of objects and events—such children's explorations become precise, apparently, only when the sighted learner has already begun to talk.

The explanation just offered is one that attributes these children's delay in speaking to lack of experience about the world. This view is distinct from the stronger claim that blind children have a special problem with conceptualization, that—as Piaget (1954) holds—concepts literally arise from motor exploration and that lack of such exploration will inevitably lead to conceptual deficit. Our data simply do not bear on this question one way or the other. They bear only on the relation between concepts and their lexical encoding: learning which word has which meaning. This learning surely requires experience of the world, for the relations between sounds and meanings are arbitrary and vary over the languages of the world. Blind learners cannot look out and see, and for some time they cannot even reach out and touch very satisfactorily. Hence they should be and are relatively late in *labelling* lexical concepts, whether or not they are late in *acquiring* the concepts.[1]

The Growth of Language in Blind Children

On any recognizable empiricist story, a mere delay in initial onset should not be the sole outcome of the lack of a visual sensorium. As we have stated, both the physical and social-contextual supports for language learning continue—throughout life—to be significantly diminished and distorted for the blind. Mountains and clouds never become observable to the hand, not even when the haptic sensorium is fully developed. Then if language growth is a more or less direct outcome of observational-interactive opportunities, one must predict extended difficulties for the blind learner, and perhaps permanent retardation. As we will now show, this is not so.

Vocabulary Growth

Vocabulary content is a prime area where differences between blind and sighted learners might be expected. Indeed, many have supposed that blind children's knowledge of objects, motion, and space would differ according to the defect in their exploratory sensorium (Fraiberg, 1977; Hermelin and O'Connor, 1982; Andersen, Dunley, and Kekelis, 1984; see Warren, 1977, for review). If they lacked such concepts, we might expect them not to utter words that encode them early, often, or appropriately.

Early semantic categories of the blind subjects

Kelli's and Carlo's earliest single word-utterances were analyzed using Nelson's (1973) categories of semantic fields, developed for the eighteen sighted children in her study. Nelson considered the first fifty words spoken by her subjects and classified these words into six categories, designed to capture the child's earliest expressed meanings. The data from Carlo and Kelli as compared to Nelson's data for sighted children are shown in Figure 2.1 and specific vocabularies of the blind children in Table 2.1.[2] In gen-

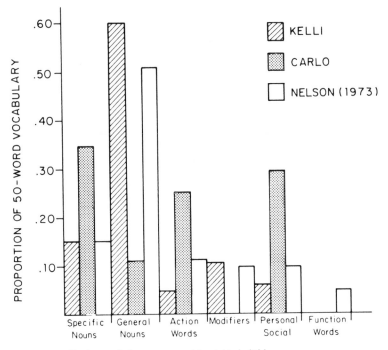

Figure 2.1 *Early vocabulary compared to sighted children*

eral, the vocabularies of the blind children appear to be the same as those of Nelson's subjects. Most of their words were specific nouns (names for people and animals), general nouns (mainly object words), and for Carlo a few numerals and personal-social words (mainly, cantankerous "No!"). Just as with sighted children at this point in development, the blind children uttered many fewer adjectives (property words) and verbs (action words) than nouns. In the major properties, then, the blind and sighted subjects exhibit the same kind of early vocabulary.

Inspecting the table and figure in detail, one finds slight differences from the sighted children. The clearest one is that in the first sample for Carlo there is a relative paucity of general nouns; however, a sample taken two months later showed a reduction in specific nouns (.16) and an increase in both general nouns (.27) and action words (.38). Hence even this one clear difference is unstable, best ascribed to sampling error (see Bigelow, 1982, for supportive evidence from other blind subjects on this topic). Further descriptive analyses that we performed achieved the same close comparability of blind children's vocabulary to that of sighted children (Landau, 1982).

Table 2.1 *Kelli's and Carlo's early vocabulary*

Kelli's first 45 words		Carlo's first 63 words	
		1st sample	2nd sample
apple cider	I burped	beep-beep	blow
babydoll	Kathy	boo-boo	button
Barbara	kitten	buck	cake
bed	kittycat	bye-bye	camera
bike	Mama	choo-choo	coffee
bird	Matt	Daddy	coin
book	meow	Diana	eat
boom	milk	down	fifty cents
car	no	five	fun
chair	nose	four	hand
cheese	pancakes	lay	he
clothes pin	pen	meow	hello
coffee	piano	Mommy	hit
cold	rubber band	money	hot
cookie monster	school	nine	in
cuckoo clock	slipper	on	Inga
Dada	smooth	one	'kay
door	Sommer	out	napkin
down	sponge	peek-boo	no
head	step	pee-you	now
hi	table	six	oh
horse	telephone	thirteen	play
	up	three	put
		tree	quarter
		T.V.	sit
		two	telephone
		up	ticky-tock
		water	touch
		toy	what
			wind
			yay
			yes
			yum

In sum, blind children talk about what most young children talk about: mommies, daddies, dolls, cookies, and toys. Our subjects' uses of such words seemed appropriate to their contexts so far as we could determine. Nothing in the later vocabulary growth of the three children supports the idea that, once speech begins, their lexicons are smaller or differ in sense from those of their sighted agemates. To the extent that such vocabulary data can be used to draw inferences about children's representations of the world, the blind children seemed to know about and be interested in the same aspects of experience as sighted children. Thus a first look at early vocabulary reveals a striking uniformity in lexical classifications despite differences in the sensorium and the information it provides. This is a beginning indication that conceptual tendencies in blind and sighted learners act to override adventitious differences in their experiential base.

Are the blind child's lexical concepts deviant or less abstract?

The conclusions just drawn contradict the position usually taken by investigators of blind children, who suppose that their linguistic concepts are deviant despite the normalcy of their initial item choices. This supposition is that the words blind and sighted children use do not refer to the world in the same way. This is an issue to which we will return in detail. For now it is worth noting that the literature on language learning in the blind often asserts that there is something distorted, meaningless, or concrete in the blind child's speech—that he uses the language superficially well but without knowing as much of what he is talking about (Cutsforth, 1951; Fraiberg, 1977; Bloom, 1983; Andersen et al., 1984). Specifically, some investigators argue that lexical items are used by blind children to refer to narrower conceptual categories than do the same items as used by sighted youngsters. The evidence adduced often comes from an alleged paucity of and different bases for "overgeneralizations" in the speech and comprehension performances of blind youngsters: that the blind do not extend lexical usage to new referents as readily as do the sighted; and that when they do, the bases for such generalizations are abnormal (Andersen et al., 1984).

Such evidence is tricky to generate or interpret, but the position is plausible enough. To the extent that certain lexical items refer to or can be interpreted—even wrongly—to refer to things in the world that resemble one another only in the visual-perceptual domain, we must expect that the blind child overgeneralizes these less than the sighted child. Why should the moon be mistaken for a ball unless one can observe the roundness of the moon—even if both the blind and the sighted child mistakenly believe that *ball* means 'round'?

The first question to be asked is whether the blind child does overgeneralize just like sighted children when the circumstances (haptic rather than visual resemblance) provide the opportunity. Quantitative evidence is hard to obtain because overgeneralization of word meaning is a much rarer phenomenon than many have thought and is restricted roughly to the first seventy-five words acquired. But we can attest to a few overgeneralizations, and these look appropriate. For example, handed a pumpkin, which she had never before observed, Kelli said "Oh, a ball."

More important, certain specifically haptic overgeneralizations characteristic of the blind might escape the notice of sighted observers, or be interpreted as bizarre, just because the sighted observer's salient organization of properties is different from that of the blind. For example, the confusability functions among the braille characters by blind children are quite surprising to a sighted observer and might easily be thought of as revealing a general incapacity to deal with abstract materials. However, recall Millar's (1978) findings on this topic from Chapter 1: Blind children do generalize systematically about these characters, but the basis for their generalizations is primarily their density rather than their spatial properties. Millar's sophisticated analysis uncovers the basis for these novel generalizations and hence credits blind children with their own nonconcreteness.

In sum, anecdotal evidence about overgeneralizations (or lack of them) is hard to interpret even in the normal sighted case. It is even harder to interpret for the blind barring a detailed inquiry about perceptual saliencies in the haptic domain. Thus, in our opinion, it is not possible to rank blind and sighted children for relative "abstractness" of thought.[3]

Syntactic growth

Similar issues pertain to patterns of syntactic growth. Here too real-world experience would seem to be a component in solving this problem, and here too the blind child might encounter difficulties (as previously mentioned in our discussion of cats on mats and mats under cats). To assess syntactic growth, we continued to observe the three subjects in informal play sessions, videotaping these observations and submitting the findings to standard descriptive analyses. The measurements begin with language onset for Kelli and Carlo, but our first session with Angie occurred when she was 29 months old. As we begin to show here, development in the blind learners is normal both in rate and in internal structure and content.

Mean utterance length

The first standard measure we used was mean length of the child's utterance in morphemes (MLU) during a single session, following the coding procedure developed by Brown (1973). For example, "Book on table" would be scored as a three-morpheme sentence; "Books on table" would be a four-morpheme sentence (book + s

+ on + table). Though evidently quite superficial, this measure is revealing just because the length of the child's sentences is a fairly direct consequence of growing competence in many important properties of the underlying linguistic system (see Brown, 1973, for a demonstration that MLU grows in an orderly way across individual children; and Shipley, Smith, and Gleitman, 1969, who showed that a closely related measure, median utterance length, correlates better with other measures of language growth than any of these other measures do with each other). Reliability checks on our coding were conducted by having an assistant not involved in the research independently code two sessions for each of the three subjects (reliability was above .9).

Figures 2.2 and 2.3 compare the blind subjects' rate of growth in MLU to those for Brown's and for Bloom, Lightbown, and Hood's (1975) sighted normal subjects on this measure. Figure 2.4 compares them to five equally premature sighted subjects studied by

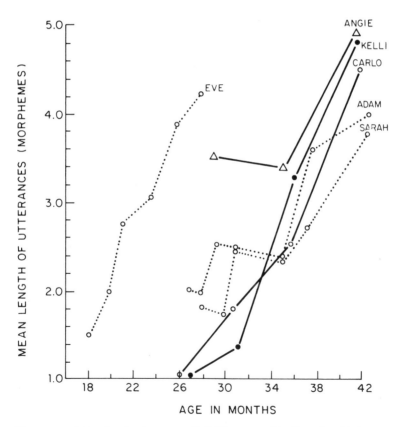

Figure 2.2 *Mean length of utterance (MLU) compared to Brown's subjects*

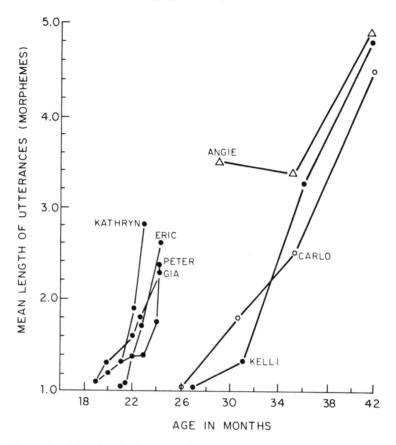

Figure 2.3 *Mean length of utterance (MLU) compared to Bloom's subjects*

us. Inspection of the figures shows an effect that seems to confirm the expectation of continued difficulty for the blind child. The first few measurements of MLU show that Carlo and Kelli are late compared to the sighted individuals in putting together two morphemes in a single sentence. As remarked in our initial sketch of these children, the first two-word utterances occurred at 29 months in Kelli and some time between 28 and 30 months in Carlo. This is later than for any of the sighted subjects studied by Brown and Bloom et al. However, again both of them fell just within the range for normal sighted children. Lenneberg (1967) reported that 50 percent of sighted full-term children produce two-word sentences by 18 months and 75 percent do so by 22 months. The Bayley norms are similar, with a mean age of 20.6 months; but again, there is a wide age range, from 16 to 30 months, just covering the blind subjects' ages of syntax onset. Our

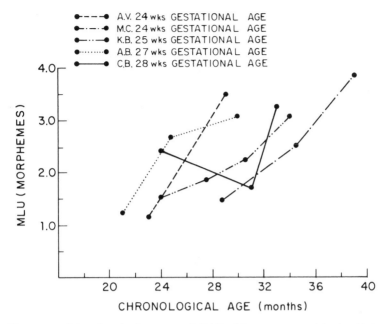

Figure 2.4 *Mean length of utterance (MLU) of five premature sighted subjects*

sighted subjects who, like Kelli and Carlo, were two to three months premature, were delayed compared to full-term children but still faster than the blind premature children.

However, these first few measurements do not index a continuing retardation but are simply the tag-end consequence of the blind subjects' relatively late language onset. Thereafter they jump in their rate of progress and rapidly catch up to their sighted full-term peers, with the MLU measures of Carlo and Kelli equal to that of Brown's Adam and Sarah by 36 months, as Figure 2.2 reveals (note that the same rapid catch-up characterizes the sighted premature population shown in Figure 2.4). As for our full-term subject, Angie, she was reported by her mother to be a very early speaker. At our first direct measurement (29 months) she already had an MLU of 3.60, more precocious than two of Brown's three subjects.

Details of the rate of MLU change were also normal for all three blind subjects. The figures show that MLU for the sighted subjects climbs from a mean of about 1.5 words to a mean of 3–3.5 words within about six to twelve months. For Bloom et al.'s subjects and for Brown's Eve, this spans ages 18 to 24 months. For Brown's other two subjects, it spans about ages 24 to 36 months. For the sighted premature subjects, it spans about ages 24 to 36 months.

For Kelli and Carlo, the period was similar, spanning 26 to 35 months. During the succeeding six months, Kelli and Carlo showed another jump, to an average utterance about 4.5 morphemes long. Roughly the same six-month growth curve was found for Brown's Adam and Sarah. Angie was above the mean at each observation point. On this measure, then, rate of development after initial speech onset was normal for the blind subjects. By the fourth birthday, both blind and sighted children achieved respectable MLU's above 4.0.

Summarizing, the two blind subjects for whom we have direct early data started late and then rapidly caught up to their sighted peers, with MLU measures normal by 36 months. At least a portion of their initial delay must be attributed to their extreme prematurity and illness during the first months of life; correcting for this, their onset was still late, though within the normal range. The third subject was precocious from the first available measurement.

Semantic-relational (thematic) organization

We next considered the expressed thematic relations in the children's early multiple-word utterances. This is the standard way of assessing compositional meaning, the appearance of predicate-argument structure in children's language. Bloom et al. (1975) codified these relations in the early language of their subjects and suggested a developmental sequence reflecting both the semantic and syntactic complexity of a given expressed relation. They found that the earliest relations were simple expressions of existence, negation, and recurrence, followed by actions and states, and finally the instrument, dative, and Wh-questions. The categories developed by these investigators may need some revision and extension as attempts are made to connect the categories uncovered by linguists to those uncovered by psychologists who work with child-language data. But the Bloom et al. categories seem a sensible first attempt, and as such have been used widely as an assessment tool. Adopting this system and controlling for linguistic level (by comparable MLU), we analyzed our subjects' language for the quality of these expressed semantic relations.

The results are shown in Figures 2.5, 2.6, and 2.7, which display successive samples for the blind children and sighted controls. Figure 2.5 shows Kelli and Carlo at MLU 1.78 and 1.77, respectively; Figure 2.6 shows these same subjects at MLU 3.25 and 2.71 respectively; and Figure 2.7 shows Angie at the first sample we collected, MLU 3.60. (Later samples from Angie and the other

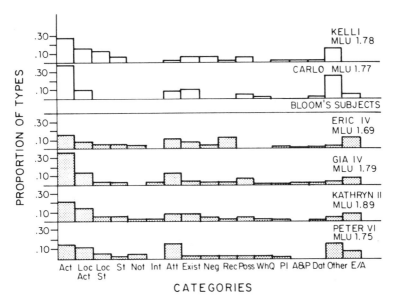

Figure 2.5 *Semantic relations in early language sample*

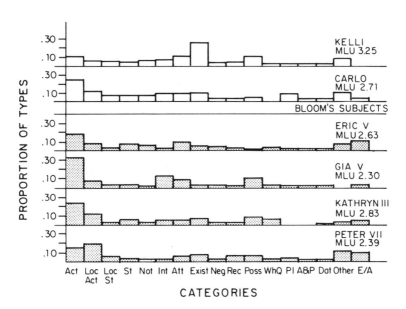

Figure 2.6 *Semantic relations in later language sample*

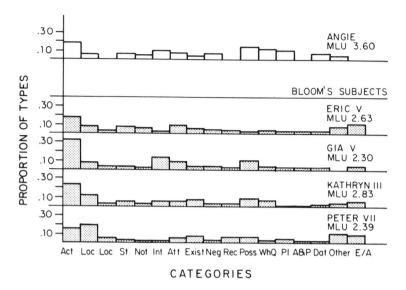

Figure 2.7 *Semantic relations in Angie's language sample*

subjects are so sophisticated as to make the current analysis inappropriate.) The control data in these figures are from Bloom et
al.'s subjects at comparable MLU levels.

Inspection of the figures reveals that the blind and sighted children are much alike. At the earliest measurement all the children
predominantly spoke about actions (both locative and nonlocative); Kelli also talked about states, as did the sighted children;
and both Kelli and Carlo talked about a smattering of other relations, such as possession, attributes, and existence, as did the
sighted children.

The differences that can be seen in the tabulated results appear
to be unstable, largely attributable to sampling error and transient
individual differences uncorrelated with the blindness. As one
example, Carlo at the first measurement (Figure 2.5) expressed a
more limited range of semantic relations than either Kelli or the
sighted children, but in the next sample taken three months later
(Figure 2.6) he expressed all relations except one (WH-question)
and in roughly the same relative proportions as Kelli, Angie, and
Bloom et al.'s subjects. As a second example, Kelli's comments
about the existence of objects (usually as pointed out to some
other person, e.g., "That's a dog") increased at the point when it
was decreasing in the sighted subjects (compare Figures 2.5 and
2.6) and then decreased. However, such an effect is not discernible

even for Carlo, the other blind subject who contributes data at the relevant time periods. Thus there are no stable deviancies discernible on these measures, characteristic of the development of blind subjects as opposed to sighted subjects.

Internal syntactic structure

Here we consider the internal complexity of the child's surface syntax; specifically, the number and complexity of noun phrases (NP) such as "the ball" and verb phrases (VP) such as "hit the bat." The coding categories follow those developed by Newport (1977), and the analyses compare her sighted subjects to our blind subjects at the same MLU levels.[4] Thus we can ask, as the blind child's sentences grow in sheer length, whether growth is in terms of the same structural parameters that characterize language growth in the sighted population.

Table 2.2 shows an analysis of the NP and VP complexity of each blind child's language at varying MLUs. Where the data exist, each sample is compared to a subset of Newport's subjects with MLUs in a narrow range covering the blind children's MLUs. The results are summarized in Table 2.3, indicating the categories on which the subjects fell within (0), outside on the lower end (−), or outside on the upper end (+) in each sample. The analysis in Table 2.4 shows the change (difference score) over six months in the blind children's language for each category considered above. (Here the number of relevant controls decreases from the last comparison; this is because a relevant sighted control must be at the appropriate MLU level at their first of two samples, in order to use a difference measure.)

It is obvious from the tabulated results that there is no general pattern of deficit. All in all, the haphazard samples of speech produced during our taping sessions show the individual blind subjects varying on the (also haphazard) samples produced during the taping sessions by Newport, sometimes exceeding the normal subjects' output on some measure, sometimes falling below it; often, on the next assessment, the comparative facts change around. Most of the differences that appear between the sighted and blind subjects in the tables are thus best ascribed to sampling error. At roughly the same linguistic level (indexed by MLU), the blind children exhibited internal complexity of speech equal to sighted children. But there is a single exception to this general finding of sameness: All the blind subjects were delayed—though not deviant—compared to the sighted subjects in the development of verb-auxiliary structure (words and inflections per verb).

Table 2.2 *Syntactic complexity of blind children's language, compared to Newport's (1977) subjects as MLU controls*

Subject/Age[a]	MLU	NPs	Wds/NP	Inf/NP
Sample I				
Kelli–29 mos.	1.88	1.13	1.14	0.00
Carlo–27 mos.	1.75	.78	1.07	0.02
Controls				
M–24 mos.	1.55	.99	1.25	.04
C–24 mos.	1.61	1.11	1.05	.27
W–24 mos.	1.74	.97	1.13	.13
T–26 mos.	2.13	1.13	1.08	.19
B–25 mos.	2.21	.93	1.24	.12
Angie–29 mos.	4.42	1.54	1.33	.31
Controls				
S–28 mos.	3.71	1.39	1.22	.27
C–31 mos.	3.78	1.40	1.34	.12
T–31 mos.	3.87	1.52	1.31	.12
Sample II				
Kelli–33 mos.	4.07	1.71	1.39	.21
Angie–35 mos.	3.97	1.58	1.31	.18
Controls				
S–28 mos.	3.71	1.39	1.22	.27
C–31 mos.	3.78	1.40	1.34	.12
T–31 mos.	3.87	1.52	1.31	.12
Carlo–32 mos.	3.33	1.32	1.23	.08
Controls				
S–21 mos.	3.32	1.14	1.35	.11
McG–28 mos.	3.44	1.38	1.24	.15
C–25 mos.	3.46	1.47	1.21	.20
W–31 mos.	3.53	1.67	1.18	.12
Sample III				
Kelli–39 mos.	5.44	1.88	1.29	.21
Carlo–39 mos.	4.89	1.66	1.29	.15
Angie–42 mos.	4.67	1.64	1.33	.24

a. Blind subjects' ages corrected for prematurity (Kelli and Carlo).
b. Words and inflections per verb with miscellaneous items (e.g., particles) included.
c. Words and inflections per verb without miscellaneous items included.

VPs	Wds/Vb[b]	Inf/Vb[b]	Wds/Vb[c]	Inf/Vb[c]
.38	1.29	.09	1.00	.10
.74	1.34	.02	1.00	.02
.20	1.13	.00	1.32	.30
.06	1.20	.00	1.22	.00
.39	1.03	.02	1.00	.02
.49	1.20	.05	1.07	.06
.59	1.39	.09	1.12	.10
.88	1.38	.52	1.06	.52
.80	1.61	.17	1.37	.18
.72	1.76	.41	1.54	.47
.79	1.74	.17	1.52	.18
.42	1.21	50	1.04	.50
.59	1.44	.34	1.20	.34
.80	1.61	.17	1.37	.18
.72	1.76	.41	1.54	.47
.79	1.74	.17	1.52	.18
.86	1.40	.33	1.00	.33
.47	1.13	.13	1.01	.15
.66	1.60	.18	1.34	.20
.65	1.48	.27	1.31	.29
.77	1.60	.06	1.37	.08
1.12	1.51	.56	1.30	.56
.97	1.66	.45	1.20	.45
.77	1.41	.60	1.22	.60

Table 2.3 *Summary of Newport analyses: blind children inside (0), outside below (−), or outside above (+) the sighted range for MLU controls (mean values for each category)*

Subject	MLU	NPs	Wds/NP	Inf/NP
Sample I				
Kelli	1.88	0	−(.04)	0
Carlo	1.75	−(.15)	0	−(.02)
Angie	4.42	+(.02)	0	+(.04)
Sample II				
Kelli	4.07	+(.19)	+(.05)	0
Carlo	3.33	0	0	−(.03)
Angie	3.97	+(.06)	0	0
Sample III[c]				
Kelli	5.44	+(.36)	0	0
Carlo	4.89	+(.14)	0	0
Angie	4.67	+(.12)	0	0

a. Words and inflections per verb with miscellaneous items (e.g. particles) included.
b. Words and inflections per verb without miscellaneous items included.

The verb-auxiliary structure

As just noted, there was one systematic exception to the pattern of normal growth of structure in the blind learners' speech. This was for growth of verb-auxiliary structure, which seems to lag consistently behind in the early years of the blind child's life, even that of the otherwise precocious child, Angie (see Table 2.3). Growth in this aspect of language is measured simply by counting the mean number of morphemes that appear in the verb + auxiliary, where *look* is counted as one morphene, *can look* or *looked* as two morphemes, and *will have looked* as four morphemes. Thus when we say the blind are delayed in this property, we mean that at the age when sighted children usually can produce constructions like "I am eating the pizza" the blind children still say "I eating the pizza."

Why should this one arcane problem show up, and what is its importance? It might be plausible to suppose that blind children have trouble learning verbs, owing to possible difficulties in observing motion in space. However, it is not the verbs themselves but rather the morphological material having to do with tense, mood, and the like (e.g., *can, will, -ed*) whose appearance is delayed, while the motion and action verbs (e.g., *go, push, get*) are

VPs	Wds/Vb[a]	Inf/Vb[a]	Wds/Vb[b]	Inf/Vb[b]
0	0	0	0	0
+(.15)	0	0	0	0
+(.08)	−(.23)	+(.11)	−(.31)	+(.05)
−(.30)	−(.40)	+(.09)	−(.33)	+(.03)
+(.09)	0	+(.05)	−(.01)	+(.04)
−(.13)	−(.17)	0	−(.17)	0
+(.32)	−(.10)	+(.15)	−(.07)	+(.09)
+(.17)	0	+(.04)	−(.17)	0
0	−(.20)	+(.19)	−(.15)	+(.13)

c. Sample III of the blind children's language is compared here to the same controls as in sample II above. This is because Newport's data do not include MLUs higher than this level.

used appropriately at the ordinary ages. To find out why this delay in verbal auxiliaries is found, and why it matters, we will take a detour to describe the role such items play in language and how they are learned.

Closed class and open class

The verbal auxiliaries are examples of so-called *closed class* words. It is this fact that explains the special properties of their learning. The morphological stock of a natural language is partitioned into this closed class and an opposing *open class*. The open class consists of the major lexical categories, noun, verb, and adjective (called open class because it changes its membership frequently—words in this group come and go over historical time, depending on what is important for the culture to name). The second class, much smaller in membership, consists of the "little" words and affixes such as determiners (*the, this, a*), personal pronouns (*him, they*), relativizers (*that, which*), connectives (*and, or*), auxiliaries (*can, may*), prepositions (*in, of*), derivational suffixes (*-ness, -ity, -ify*), inflectional suffixes (*-ed, -en, -s*), etc. (the closed class, so called because its membership is quite resistant to language change.

Table 2.4 *Rate of growth in syntax (Newport analyses), for two six-month growth periods*

Subject	NPs	Wds/NP	Inf/NP
Growth period			
Sample I–II			
Kelli	.58	.25	.21
Carlo	.54	.16	−.06
Angie[c]	.04	−.02	−.13
Controls[d]			
(for Kelli and Carlo)			
M	.46	−.01	.19
C	.32	.12	−.10
W	.70	.05	−.01
Sample II–III			
Kelli	.17	−.10	.00
Carlo	.34	.06	.07
Angie	.06	.02	.06
Controls			
(for Carlo)			
S	.25	−.13	.16
C	−.07	.13	−.08

a. Words and inflections per verb with miscellaneous items (e.g. particles) included.
b. Words and inflections per verb without miscellaneous items included.
c. Angie began at a higher level than controls on all but the category Wds/Vb without miscellaneous items included.
d. Control data were only available for some subjects during some growth peri-

This partitioning of the morphemes turns out to be relevant to many aspects of language form and function. Because the open-closed class distinction is simply a collapsing of the lexical form-class distinction (nouns, verbs, and adjectives as against all other classes), it is obvious that the relative distribution of these items in sentences—where they can and cannot appear in constructions—differs too. For related reasons, the closed-class items are restricted in the semantic functions they subserve (nobody's name is a preposition). In languages such as English and many others, the closed class is also phonologically distinctive. Closed-class items are unstressed in most syntactic positions, deform in their phonetic content depending on their phonological and syntactic positions in sentences, and often contract ("I have been looking

VPs	Wds/Vb[a]	Inf/Vb[a]	Wds/Vb[b]	Inf/Vb[b]
.04	−.08	.41	.04	.40
.12	.06	.31	.00	.31
−.27	.06	−.18	.14	−.18
.55	.50	.27	.56	.30
.41	.19	.11	.35	.13
.38	.57	.04	.31	.06
.70	.30	.06	.26	.06
.11	.26	.12	.20	.12
.18	−.03	.26	.02	.26
.33	.48	.04	.30	.03
.07	.28	.14	.00	.18

ods. This was because, in order to qualify as a control, the (sighted) subjects had to have an MLU of the same level for the first sample considered, *as well as* a sample taken 6 months after that first sample. Most of Newport's subjects had their highest MLU level equivalent to only the first sample of the blind subjects; hence no second sample was available.

him for hours" may come out something like "I've been lookin' frim frours").

There is abundant evidence that the two classes are distinct in how they are treated during the processing of sentences. For example, Garrett (1975) showed that speech errors that are reversals (saying "Older men prefer to tend younger women" when "Older men tend to prefer younger women" was intended) switch within open-class items but not between an open and closed class item (an error like "Older men to tend prefer younger women" rarely if ever occurs). Another indication of the differences in how these classes are processed is their independent dissolution in language pathologies (Marin, Saffran, and Schwartz, 1976; Kean, 1979). Loss of the closed class in speech is the very hallmark of Broca's aphasia, while radical loss of open-class vocabulary characterizes anomia and Wernicke's aphasia.[5]

Of fundamental interest in the present context is that these two classes also differ in the patterns by which they are learned. The closed class is acquired late relative to the open class and in a distinctive developmental pattern by all youngsters learning English (Brown, 1973). Why should this be? The first guess at an answer has to do with the semantic factors we have discussed above. After all, nouns, verbs, and adjectives refer to things, events, and properties, while the closed-class items largely modulate these semantic functions and play formal syntactic roles. But this semantic explanation is hard to defend because the closed class is not equally difficult to learn in all languages. For instance, while items in this class appear late in the speech of English, Russian, and Serbo-Croatian speakers (Slobin, 1982), they appear quite early in such languages as Quiche Mayan (Pye, 1983), Turkish (Slobin, 1982), and Hebrew (Levy, 1983a).

What accounts for these crosslinguistic patterns? As Gleitman and Wanner (1982, 1984) have described, the developmental facts are adequately handled by considering the *phonological* properties of the closed class. As we stated earlier, the closed-class items are in English (and Russian and Serbo-Croatian) unstressed in most of their syntactic positions. But in Mayan and Turkish the words that fulfill the closed-class syntactic and semantic functions are usually stressed. According to Gleitman and Wanner, this difference in stress holds the key to the timing of closed-class learning: The unstressed properties of the linguistic signal are not salient to infants and very young children, who therefore omit them in speech and have trouble analyzing them for the sake of comprehension (Shipley, Smith, and Gleitman, 1969). It is in terms of just this distinction of stress that we will be able to understand the special problem of blind learners acquiring the English verbal auxiliary. To see how, we next consider the spectrum of verbal auxiliary appearance—stressed and unstressed—in English sentences.

Most auxiliary uses are unstressed just because all the auxiliary items are members of the closed class. Particularly, the auxiliary elements are unstressed and contracted in over 90 percent of declarative sentences uttered by mothers to their young sighted children (the format of "She'll eat those daisies" is preferred to that of "She will eat those daisies"; Bellugi, 1967). Yet there are special syntactic conditions under which the auxiliary cannot be contracted and usually receives stress as a function of sentential prosody. One important case occurs in yes-no questions such as

"Will she eat those daisies?" (compare *"Ll she eat those daisies?," an ungrammatical and therefore nonoccurring alternative).

If young children are especially attentive to stressed elements, as Gleitman and Wanner suppose, then they ought to learn the auxiliaries best from these stressed uses in questions and related structures. Indeed, Newport, Gleitman, and Gleitman (1977; see Furrow, Nelson, and Benedict, 1979, for a replication) showed that the frequency of yes-no questions in mothers' speech correlated positively and very strongly (on the order of .8, even after partialing to correct for initial baseline differences among the learners) with the rate of growth of the closed-class auxiliary items in young learners of English. (Also, frequency of imperatives correlated negatively with development of the auxiliary, not surprising because imperatives often lack an auxiliary.[6])

Thus mothers (of sighted children) who were disposed to use yes-no questions with high frequency had offspring who learned the auxiliary material the soonest.[7]

Learning of the verbal auxiliary by blind subjects

We can now return to the question of why the blind subjects were delayed in acquisition of the English verbal auxiliary. We analyzed the speech of Kelli's and Carlo's mothers to see whether the same relationships between maternal yes-no questions and rate of verb-auxiliary growth could account for the blind children's slowness in this single area (as for many of the other tests, our observations of Angie began too late to perform this analysis for her). As Table 2.5 shows, the two mothers' child-directed speech contains an unusually high proportion of imperatives and a very low proportion of yes-no questions, compared to Newport et al.'s means for sighted mothers. Kekelis and Andersen (1984) report the same relative frequency of imperatives in maternal speech to their blind subjects. Thus the same explanation—paucity of yes-no questions, preponderance of imperatives—that predicts late acquisition of verbal auxiliaries by sighted children of certain mothers explains the same lateness for the blind subjects.

In short, the cause of delay has to do with specific syntactic properties of the input speech to the blind rather than with constraints on inputs available to interpretation by the blind. The growth of the verbal auxiliary is certainly a function of context. But the context it is a function of is *linguistic*, not *extralinguistic*. The blind child is delayed in rate of growth on this one language dimension just because caregivers of the blind tend not to provide the optimal syntactic information.

A question remains: Why do mothers of the blind subjects

Table 2.5 *Maternal language to sighted and blind children*

Sentence type	Sighted subjects	Same age as sighted subjects		Same MLU as sighted subjects	
		Kelli	Carlo	Kelli	Carlo
Grammatical sentences					
Total grammatical	.60	.69	.63	.61	.63
Declaratives	.37	.43	.25	.25	.22
Yes-no questions	.23	.06	.14	.15	.12
Imperatives	.18	.43	.54	.45	.38
Wh-questions	.22	.08	.07	.15	.28
Other					
Total other	.40	.31	.37	.39	.37
Sentence fragments	.42	.39	.27	.38	.19
Interjections	.48	.61	.62	.46	.51
Dysfluencies	.00	.00	.03	.03	.30
Unanalyzable	.10	.00	.08	.13	.00

Note: Data for sighted children are from Newport et al. (1977). Same age data are for Kelli's and Carlo's mothers when the children were the same age as Newport et al.'s subjects. Same MLU data are for Kelli's and Carlo's mothers when the children were at the same linguistic level as Newport et al.'s subjects. Two samples were needed, since maternal language does vary with the age of the subject, and Kelli and Carlo were always older than Newport et al.'s subjects, at the same linguistic level.

Newport scored deictics separately, but we have included them in the relevant categories in this table; for example, deictic declaratives are included in the declarative category, deictic Wh-questions are included in the Wh-question category, etc.

make this unusual set of choices among the structures of the language they use in talking to their children? The answer is simple. As Newport et al. showed, mothers of normal children do not select syntactic types in a deliberate attempt to teach their offspring the niceties of grammatical structure. Rather, their aims reflect their social interactions with their offspring, and the syntactic forms of their utterances follow directly from these aims. Since the mother wants the child to drink his orange juice or pick up his blocks, she is likely to use many imperative forms and fewer declaratives. The same situational factors will be exaggerated for mothers of blind children. These youngsters often do not know what is going on in the invisible scene around them and thus can rarely be asked for information (the felicitous occasion for the yes-no question structure). They must often be told what to do and how to do it (the felicitious occasion for the imperative structure). But these very choices, sensible on social-interactive grounds, have been shown to delay acquisition of the verbal auxiliary structure in sighted children and of course have the same effect for blind children.

Summary

We found two differences in the pattern of development of blind and sighted children. The first had to do with the moment of speech onset. Normative studies had suggested that there is probably some delay in speech onset characteristic of even neurologically intact blind children, though effects of prematurity account for some of this delay. Consistent with this picture, our two premature blind children began to talk late, though just within the normal range for sighted individuals (though Angie's evident precocity suggests that late language onset, while a frequent and characteristic concomitant of blindness, is not the *necessary* outcome.) The second difference we observed was a delay in acquisition of the verbal auxiliary.

For both these features of the blind children's learning, we assigned the delay to environmental circumstances. For the onset delay, we suggested that exploration of the extralinguistic context which accompanies speech events is restricted for the blind during the first year of life because of the late appearance of haptic exploratory skills. (Though this is not, strictly speaking, an environmental circumstance, it so functions because it is a maturational effect that temporarily restricts access to the environment for the blind.) In discussing the relatively slow growth of the verbal auxiliary, we showed that the blind learners' problem derives from the special linguistic environment offered to them: Mothers ask few questions of their blind offspring and give them many commands. These speech properties, in turn, correlate with rate of appearance of the auxiliary structure for blind and sighted children alike.[8]

Over and above these differences, we are struck by the normalcy of the blind child's language development on all the other measures we have taken. The two populations are essentially indistinguishable from each other by the third birthday, including internal organization of syntax, thematic relations, and vocabulary. It seems to us remarkable that children who confront the real world as differently as blind and sighted children come to have so similar a perspective on it, as revealed by this first descriptive look at their language learning. Radically different sensory-perceptual bases for induction yield a similar pattern of language development, suggesting difficulties for any simple experiential account of such learning. These difficulties will magnify as we consider the semantics of perceptual verbs and adjectives as used by the blind.

3 / The Meaning of Sighted Verbs: *Look* as the Blind Child Applies It to Herself

The word 'statue' may be explained to a blind man by other words, when 'picture' cannot, his senses having given him the idea of figure, but not of colours, which therefore words cannot excite in him.

(John Locke, 1690, Book 3.IV.11)

So far we have been concerned only with very general properties of language growth in the blind child, and for these the picture was one of normalcy. Thus at least a start was made toward answering the first question raised in Chapter 1: Does blindness necessarily predict major delays and deficits for the language learner? We found that it does not. Here we begin to ask our second question: Do the blind have particular difficulties with just that aspect of language learning that specifically concerns the visual experience? Locke, as cited above, made predictions concerning what can and cannot be understood by a congenitally blind individual. Because the blind are assumed to be able to detect shape, they can acquire the meaning of *statue* through haptic exploration or through a verbal description whose terms are haptic-spatial. But two-dimensional representations, differentiated only through differing hues and brightnesses, can be perceived only through vision. Moreover, according to Locke, since the underlying properties—the hues and brightnesses themselves—are "simple" and thus not subject to definition by other words, no verbal description of pictures would suffice for a blind man to understand the word *picture.*

We follow Locke in supposing that a particular subset of the normal vocabulary will be the most informative in assessing the contribution of experience to language learning. In the worst case, certain lexical particulars receive no contextual-situational correlations in the blind observer's experience. Primarily these have to do with sight-related terms: verbs such as *look*, nouns such as *photograph*, and adjectives such as *green*. If some here-and-now context is required for the learning of such items, how can blind individuals ever acquire them?

Surprisingly, though, it has been noted that blind individuals do come to use these sight-related terms spontaneously. They do say *look, see, watch,* and so forth. The clinical literature on the blind has responded to this fact much in the tradition attributed to Locke. It takes for granted that blind learners cannot surmount their sensory deficits in acquiring these linguistic concepts and categories and thus assumes that their utterances of *look* or *green* are necessarily empty or meaningless—mere "verbalisms." Parents of the blind are counseled not to encourage their children to use such terms, for it can lead to "loose thinking" (Cutsforth, 1951; Tetzchner and Martinsen, 1980; and for review, Warren, 1977).

We studied two subdomains of the sight-related vocabulary, visual verbs (such as *look*) and visual adjectives (the color terms, see Chapter 8). As we will show, the young blind learner, Kelli, achieves significant understanding and use of such words. Here we ask how Kelli used *look* to refer to her own perceptual explorations, as early as her third birthday. In Chapter 4 we will ask how Kelli interpreted the two visual terms, *look* and *see*, as they refer to the perceptual activities and explorations of sighted people. Chapter 5 will discuss Kelli's spontaneous production of sighted verbs, both of herself and of others.

Subjects

The subjects for this work were Kelli at age three years, and four sighted youngsters of the same age who served as controls.

Kelli

Kelli was the sole blind subject we had the opportunity to study in these comprehension studies. She first used the words *look* and *see* in our presence at about age 28 months (see Chapter 5 for these spontaneous speech data), the normal time for appearance of such words in the sighted population as well (Bloom et al., 1975). By age 36 months, she was using these terms freely and frequently in conversation, in ways that seemed appropriate—except that we knew she was blind. At this time we began to study her comprehension of the verb *look*. Though results from a single individual cannot be applied without caution to the blind population at large, certain factors do suggest that Kelli is a fair representative of the young blind population. She was in the bottom quartile of linguistic-developmental rate for intact blind children, so she does not seem to have an especially remarkable linguistic talent. Her background is middle-class nonprofessional, so her circumstances do not set her apart in special ways. And her parents did not avail themselves of clinicians or social workers in rearing her, so no unusual tutorial situation existed during the period of investigation. It is also of some interest that the parents of other blind children with whom we are in contact report the same interpretations and spontaneous uses of visual terms that are documented more formally here for Kelli.

On the other hand, Kelli's family was unusual in their emotional acceptance of her blindness, including (as she matured) discussion of that blindness, and in their attempt to make the world understandable by engaging in games and conversation that allowed Kelli to come into tactile contact with many of the things that figured in conversation. Also, Kelli's family began from the sure belief that she would develop as a normal child; this explains why they allowed us to conduct certain experiments in which we demanded of a blind child that she "look" (similar questions are asked about the verb *see* in the next chapter). From Fraiberg's (1977) evidence and observations of a population of blind children, there is some reason to expect deficits in less favorable familial circumstances than Kelli's. Still Kelli provides evidence for the understanding that can in principle be attained by a young blind child if unfavorable situational factors do not add to the burden of learning.

The sighted children

Four sighted children of Kelli's age (33–42 months) participated in the same experiments while blindfolded. This means that both Kelli and these sighted but blindfolded children had to perform certain acts on command ("Look up!"), even though none was in a position to look, at least in the visual interpretation of that term. In this sense, the experimental situation equalized Kelli and her sighted agemates. But the control children were different from Kelli in the conditions that obtained before testing, those conditions that presumably led to the original learning of terms such as *look*.

The Hypotheses To Be Tested

Put most generally, our question was whether Kelli had acquired a meaningful interpretation of *look* that could apply to herself. As for the control children, the question was whether the interpretation they had already acquired would naturally extend to circumstances in which their vision was blocked. Depending on the answers to these questions, specific findings should be expected:

(1) If *look* is a purely visual word, then neither Kelli nor blindfolded sighted children ought to be able to respond coherently to the command "Look!" when their eyes are barred from participation. Kelli would fail both because she does not understand *look* and because she cannot see; the sighted controls would fail because they do understand *look* and because they are in a situation in which they cannot see.

(2) If *look* is a word that centrally refers to the visual experience but can be extended metaphorically by those who learned it from hearing it spoken in situations to which its visual interpretation is apposite, then the sighted children but not Kelli might be expected to respond systematically to "Look!" even when their eyes are covered.

(3) In direct contrast, if Kelli learned the word *look* but learned it differently owing to the lack of a visual sensorium, she like the sighted children should respond systematically when commanded "Look!" but her responses would differ from those of the sighted controls.

(4) Finally, if the learning of *look* and its stored sense is somehow more general and pertains to more than visual looking—perhaps being amodal—then both Kelli and the sighted children should have an interpretation for *look*, perhaps the same interpretation. In that case responses to "Look!" in the absence of visual stimulation might be expected to be the same for Kelli and the sighted children.

Plan of the Comprehension Studies

We know that sighted children explore the world predominantly by eye and that blind children explore predominantly by hand (though, to be sure, sighted children can also explore manually, and there is a panoply of ancillary haptic kinesthetic means by which blind youngsters can interact with the world outside their bodies). Therefore, at first guess, a word like *touch* or *feel* might serve for blind youngsters as *look* does for sighted children. Our aim was to discover Kelli's (and controls') glosses for the words *look* and *touch*. To do so, we tried to elicit the children's character-istic responses to requests that required observable action.

Such actions cannot, it is true, be interpreted as direct indica-tors of the meaning of the terms to their users. This is simply a fact about how words and sentences relate to the world. Particu-larly, responses to requests and commands are often affected by conversational inferences about the intent of the interlocutor that go beyond the literal meaning of words and syntactic structures (Searle, 1975; Grice, 1975). As one example, children asked to "find X" will often find it, but then give it to the interlocutor. This does not mean they don't understand *find*, but rather that they as-sume an intention that goes beyond what was said, i.e., that some-one asked one to find something because he wanted it given to him. Far be it from us to complain of these inference-based acts—without them, communication would be even harder than it is. Nevertheless, such complications pose an interpretive diffi-culty for the investigator if he is trying to determine the compo-nent lexical or syntactic functioning of child subjects. But despite these difficulties in using the child's actions to reconstruct his meanings, the experiments now to be reported achieved system-atic, but different, responses from Kelli and the sighted children. Moreover, the responses also differed systematically as a function of the verb (*look* or *touch*) in each command.[1]

An important detail for interpreting the results has to do with the order in which the experiments were carried out. For Kelli, the reader can easily reconstruct the order by noting her age at the time of each experiment. For the sighted children, the order of presentation of the experiments was systematically varied among the four subjects. This is crucial because they might have been learning something in one of the experiments that they used to understand how to behave in the next. As it turned out, the pre-sentation order had no particular effect.

Experiment 1: Does look mean 'touch' to the blind child?

Setting. In this experiment and all that follow, Kelli and the sighted control children were tested individually in their homes or a laboratory room familiar to them during informal play periods. The experimenter gave the subject a command and waited for a response. Usually the children responded immediately; if they did not, the command was repeated. No child failed to respond after two such presentations of a command. The closest pacing of pre-sentation of commands was one minute but often much slower, sometimes as far apart as thirty minutes. All sessions were videotaped. The analysis of the results was always based on the video-taped behaviors.

Subjects. Kelli was 36 months old when this experiment was conducted. The four sighted blindfolded controls ranged in age from 33 to 42 months.

Stimuli and procedure. The subjects were presented with the commands to *Look up, Look down, Look behind you, Look in front of you, Look over here by me,* and *Look over there by Mommy.* These commands were in the single order listed above to all subjects. The contexts varied: Some commands were presented when no object was in the target location (e.g., *Look up,* when no object was in the space above the subject's body), and others were presented when an object (a graduated ring tower) was in the target location (e.g., *Look behind you,* when the ring tower had been placed behind the subject's body). When there was an object in the location mentioned, sometimes the child was made aware of this and sometimes not.

Coding. Here, as for all succeeding procedures, the videotaped behaviors, including the subject's verbal responses, were coded by the experimenter or an assistant in terms of the relevant variables (e.g., 'orients head toward,' 'contacts with the hand'). Sample reliability checks for all coding procedures (for these and for the further procedures to be reported) were made by an independent observer and were in each case at or above .90.

Results. The contextual circumstances (whether or not an object was at the target location or known to be there in advance) had no effect on the responses of the subjects. Blindness versus blindfoldedness, in contrast, resulted in responses so distinct as to require no tabular presentation. Kelli moved her hands in the appropriate spatial directions (that is, up, down, and so on), usually exploring to find if there was something there but *never* tilting her head to face the object, in six out of six trials. Her head remained facing forward, even when she was responding to "Look behind you." In clear contrast, each blindfolded sighted child moved her head in the appropriate spatial directions (e.g., tilting the head up to "Look up") in six out of six trials. Figures 3.1 and 3.2 show examples of these behaviors.

This different pattern of response for blind and sighted subjects is significant ($p = .001$, Fisher exact test). A satisfactory first gloss is that *look* means 'turn one's eyes toward' for a sighted child (though 'turn one's nose toward' or 'orient the face toward' would do as well) while *look* means 'contact with the hands' to the blind child.

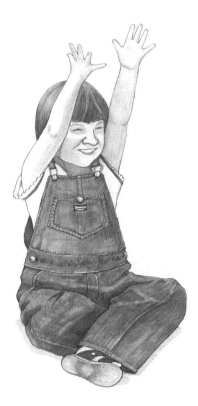

Figure 3.1 *Kelli's response to "look up!" In Experiment 1, the blind child moved her hands, not her eyes and head, in the direction indicated by the command in six out of six trials.*

Experiment 2: Look *is more like 'apprehend' to the blind child*

The results of Experiment 1 might simply mean that for Kelli *look* meant 'touch.' But this interpretation runs up against a problem. For in fact Kelli almost never used the (known) word *touch* that, in the speech of her mother, coded precisely the meaning she allegedly had in mind for her own haptic activities. So we next tried to find out whether *look* was distinct from *touch* for Kelli.

Our first approach was to pit these two words against each other. When told "Touch X but don't look at it," Kelli would usually simply touch or stroke the object or bang it with her fist. Then told "Now you can look at it," she would manually explore

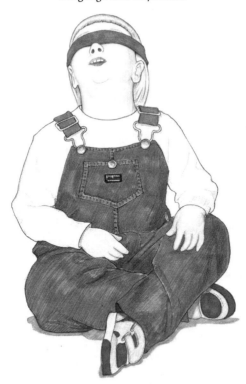

Figure 3.2 *A blindfolded sighted child's response to "look up!" In Experiment 1, each child moved her eyes and head, not her hands, in the direction indicated by the command in six out of six trials.*

it extensively, running her hands over all its surfaces (see Landau, 1982, for the full results of this procedure).

We next asked whether certain adjectival and adverbial modifications of *look* produce still more distinctive behaviors. We reasoned that responses to, e.g., "look very hard" and "touch very hard" might be more distinguishable from one another than simply "look" and "touch." As will now be shown, the pattern of results strongly suggests a distinction between these two verbs as Kelli construed them.

Subjects. This experiment was also performed when Kelli was 36 months, but a couple of weeks older than she was during Experiment 1. The four blindfolded sighted children ranged from 33 to 42 months.

Stimuli and procedure. Using several toys, we asked Kelli to "look" or "touch" (1) with spatial modifiers: *up, behind you, in that* (container), *under* (some object), and *here*; (2) with intensity modifiers: *real hard, gently, real good*; and (3) with instruments of contact or perception: *with your finger, foot, nose, mouth, ear.* For each of these modifiers two commands were given, one using *look* and the other using *touch.* For example, a pair of intensity commands was "Look at (object) gently" and "Touch (object) gently." This yielded a total of twenty-six commands (thirteen pairs), presented in a randomized order over three experimental sessions.

The sighted blindfolded children were tested for a subset of these stimuli, namely *behind you, up, with your foot, finger, mouth, nose, ear.* This yielded a total of fourteen commands (seven pairs), presented in a randomized order within a single session.

Analysis. The behavioral descriptions were first coded for whether or not the member of a pair (*look* and *touch*) elicited different responses or the same response (*differentiated* versus *not differentiated* in Tables 3.1 and 3.3 for the blind and sighted subjects, respectively). Next all the responses for Kelli were coded as to whether they were *exploratory* or *nonexploratory*, as summarized in Table 3.2. For example, extensive manipulation of an object with examination of all its parts was called an exploratory response; banging the object with closed fist was called nonexploratory. While these two categories could be used to organize all but one

Table 3.1 *Experiment 2:* Look *is more like "apprehend" to the blind child (Kelli's behavior)*

Command types	Look	Touch
Differentiated		
up	nonexploratory	exploratory
behind you	exploratory	nonexploratory
real hard	exploratory	nonexploratory
gently	exploratory	nonexploratory
with finger	exploratory	nonexploratory
with foot	exploratory	nonexploratory
with nose	exploratory	nonexploratory
with mouth	exploratory	nonexploratory
Nondifferentiated		
under	exploratory(?)[a]	exploratory(?)
in the X	exploratory	other
real good	nonexploratory	nonexploratory
with ear	exploratory(?)	exploratory(?)
here	exploratory	exploratory

a. For those marked (?) there was some doubt as to the classification. For instance, asked to look for something "under the table," she put her head down under the table and then asked for the object, "Can I have X?" But notice that these coding questions only arise among the nondifferentiated command types.

Table 3.2 *Experiment 2: Summary of Kelli's behavioral types (exploratory/non-exploratory) in response to two verbs* (look/touch)

Behavior	Look	Touch	Total
Exploratory	11	4	15
Nonexploratory	2	8	10

of Kelli's responses without coding difficulty, the response styles of the sighted subjects were quite different and required different coding categories that we will describe later (Table 3.3).

Results and discussion

Responses of Kelli. Inspection of Table 3.1 reveals that for eight of the thirteen command types (*up, behind you, real hard, gently, with your finger, foot, nose, mouth*), Kelli distinguished between *touch* and *look* command pairs. For the remaining five command types (*under, in the container, real good, with your ear, here*), Kelli behaved no differently for *look* versus *touch* commands, sometimes exploring and sometimes touching for each.

For the eight command types among which Kelli differentiated, the interpretive distinction is very clear. She consistently (seven out of eight trials) interpreted *touch* as 'contact' (bang, scratch, tap); *look* was never interpreted this way in eight trials. In contrast, *look* was consistently interpreted as 'explore' or 'apprehend' (manipulate, feel all over, pretend to eat or smell): seven of eight commands to "look" elicited exploratory responses.

A few examples will make this pattern clearer (see also Figure 3.3). In response to "look behind you," Kelli searched around in the area behind her with her hands, but when told to "touch behind you" she touched her back. When told to "look real hard" she rubbed the object all over, running her hand along its surfaces; when told to "touch real hard" she banged her hand against the object. Thus *touch* and *look* are distinguished by whether or not they elicit exploratory behavior. Two of Kelli's responses may hint that her interpretation of *look* is not restricted to manual exploration but may extend to any exploratory behavior. Told to "look with your mouth" she pretended to taste (held it up to her mouth), but asked to "touch with your mouth" she bent down and pressed her mouth against the object; told to "look with your nose" she sniffed at the object, but told to "touch with your nose" she bent her head down and pressed her nose against it. In general, for all differentiated responses, each response to *look* was

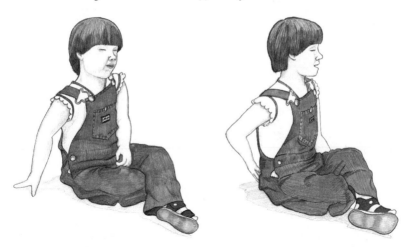

Figure 3.3 *Kelli's response to "look behind you" (a) and "touch behind you" (b). In Experiment 2, the blind child responded differentially to commands modifying* look *vs commands modifying* touch.

made by moving the object to the named organ; each response to *touch* was made by moving the named organ to the object.

Thus Kelli differentiated between commands to look and commands to touch. To evaluate these results statistically, we tabulated her responses to all the stimulus commands, including the pairs where her behavior was not differentiated for *look* versus *touch*. Table 3.2 thus organizes the *exploratory/nonexploratory* responses as a function of the *look/touch* commands (omitting one uncodable response). The pattern of differentiation between *look* and *touch* commands is highly significant (p < .025, Fisher exact test).

Responses of the sighted children. The results for the sighted blindfolded subjects are shown in Table 3.3. These children also usually (a mean of 9.6 of the fourteen commands) differentiated between *look* and *touch* commands. The predominant response to *touch* was simple manual contact; the predominant response to *look* was "visual," as described more fully below. The comparison of these contact responses and visual responses to the two verbs is statistically significant (Chi Square = 22.94, df = 1, p < .01).

In detail, the response types, where differentiated, were in some ways similar to Kelli's. The predominant interpretation of *touch* was a simple manual contact (3.5 of 4.8), while *look* was infrequently interpreted this way (0.8 of 4.8). But the responses to the *look* commands were altogether different from Kelli's. Most fre-

Table 3.3 *Experiment 2: Mean responses to* look *versus* touch *by sighted children*

Behavior	Look	Touch	Total
Did differentiate	4.8	4.8	9.6
Manual			
Exploratory	0.0	0.3	0.3
Nonexploratory (contact)	0.8	3.5	4.3
Orients hands only	0.0	0.3	0.3
"*Visual*"			
Orients head only	2.5	0.0	2.5
Orients head plus hand movement	0.3	0.7	1.0
Makes analogy to vision	1.2	0.0	1.2
Did not differentiate	2.2	2.2	4.4
Total	7.0	7.0	14.0

quently, commands to *look* seemed to be interpreted as commands to do something visual (with the eyes), even though the eyes were covered: The children oriented their heads in the direction indicated by the command. The second most frequent response was to do something we called "analogy to vision." Here they behaved as though the organ named could see (be used as a distance receptor), orienting that organ toward the object (e.g., bringing the foot close to but not touching the object). Finally, there was occasionally some additional activity accompanying the visual responses (orientation of eyes) whose sense we could not decipher: The child would orient the head as if to look at something but also, e.g., turn the head from side to side (for examples of these behaviors, see Figure 3.4 and the figure at note 2 to this chapter).

In sum, the sighted children understood *look* only when it could be interpreted as a visual experience. Since they were blindfolded in this experiment, they settled for orienting their covered eyes in the direction of the named object or (so it seemed to us), pretending that a named organ had grown an eye and orienting *this* in the direction of the named object. In contrast, they interpreted *touch* to mean 'contact.' Recall that Kelli also distinguished *look* from *touch* on a considerable number of commands. But her response to *look* was never a mere orientation of the named "sensor." Rather, when *look* and *touch* were differentiated, the former was most often interpreted as 'explore' and the latter as 'contact.'

Our preliminary conclusion is that *look* is tied to the visual modality for the sighted children, while *touch* is interpreted as physical contact. For Kelli, too, *touch* implies physical contact. But from

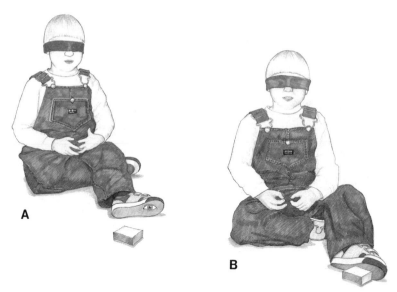

Figure 3.4 *A blindfolded sighted child's response to "look with your foot" (a) and "touch with your foot" (b). In Experiment 2, the blindfolded sighted children made "visual" responses to* look *commands, for example by behaving as though the named instrument could perceive at a distance. In contrast, they made contact responses to* touch *commands.*

the evidence presented so far, one might suspect that for her *look* means 'to perceive and apprehend, independent of modality.' This interpretation would explain her responses to "look with the nose" as sniffing and "look with the mouth" as pretending to taste. It is important in this context to note that the sighted children's visual analogies were not at all like Kelli's responses to *look*. They did not seem to assume that the foot and nose could "look" in the sense that they are exploratory sensoria, albeit not really visual ones. Rather they seemed to assume that—given the bizarre situation—their feet or noses had grown an eye, which, hypothetically or metaphorically speaking, could look—visually, in the way the eye looks, by orienting the line of sight and perceiving at a distance.

But establishing the sense of these words for the blind and sighted children required further inquiry. We had to find out (Experiments 3 and 4) whether Kelli distinguished looking from other perceptions (such as listening), so as to determine whether the item *look* meant 'apprehend by any modality,' as just suggested, or was specific to the haptic modality. After all, only two of many commands suggested that *look* might for her have had an amodal interpretation. And we had to find out (Experiment 5) whether the sighted blindfolded children could be induced to "look" with their hands, in which case we might have to revise the conjecture that their use of the item *look* is specific to vision.

Experiment 3:
Do all perceptual verbs mean 'explore haptically'?

Stimuli and procedure. In this probe, conducted when Kelli was 39 months, she was given commands to "look at," "touch," "listen to," and "taste" various objects. She was given three of each kind of command, using overlapping but not identical objects across command types. Some of these were natural ("Look at the orange ring"), some unnatural ("Taste the radio"), and some were in between in plausibility ("Listen to the orange ring," said as the experimenter tapped that ring to produce a sound). The twelve commands were randomized and presented every so often during the session. But one command was inadvertently omitted, leaving eleven responses.

Results and discussion. Kelli was appropriately discriminating, responding according to the verb in the command for 10 of the 11 stimuli, a statistically significant difference between appropriate and inappropriate responses ($p = .005$, Binomial Test). (The discordant response to "listen to the raisins," though possibly appropriate, was hard to evaluate and thus scored as incorrect: First she sat still, then reached out, saying "raisins"). When asked to "touch" or "look at" objects, she reached out and took them. When asked to "listen to" some object, she became quiet and oriented her head to the sound but did not move toward it. When asked to "taste" an object, she licked it, even if it was inedible. For examples of these behaviors, see Figure 3.5. It seems that *look* is interpreted as calling for haptic exploration, while other specific verbs are used for apprehension by other means.

Experiment 4: Does look mean 'perceive by any modality'?

To determine whether *look* biased Kelli to explore an object manually rather than to explore by any reasonable perceptual means, we created a situation obverse to that in Experiment 3. This time Kelli was always asked to "look," never to "listen." But the situations varied in how plausible it would be to explore by hand. For instance, the plausible way to perceive a radio playing at a distance (given the real uses of radios) is by listening to it. Thus if

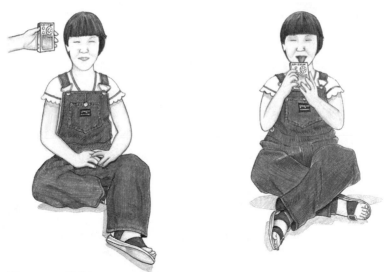

Figure 3.5 *Kelli's response to "listen to the radio" and "taste the radio." In Experiment 3, the blind child differentiated among the perceptual verbs by responding differently to commands to* look, touch, listen, *and* taste. *She responded appropriately on ten of eleven commands.*

Kelli thought *look* meant 'perceive, modality independent,' we might expect her just to listen when told to "look at the radio" when it was far away and playing, just as she previously had quieted and oriented her head when asked to "listen" in Experiment 3. To model this idea, we varied the perceptual information available at the time of the command. Kelli was 37 months old when this experiment was done.

Setting and materials. Kelli was asked to "look" at various objects, under three conditions of available perceptual information. Each of these objects could in principle be contacted manually, explored manually, or heard (such objects as a radio and a squeaking toy fish were used). In the *tactile* condition, Kelli's hand was placed on the object just as the command was given; in two of four such presentations, the object was behind her body, and in the other half it was in front. In the *aural* condition, Kelli was not touching the object, but it was sounded as the command was given. On two of four trials the object was far from Kelli (about eight feet away), and in the other two trials it was quite close to her (within arm's reach). In the *visual* condition, Kelli could not perceive the object at all as the command was given: It was not in her hand and it was not making any noise (the radio was off, the fish wasn't squeaking). Again, in two of four instances, the object was far from Kelli, and in two instances it was close to her.

Results and discussion. What should we expect the results to be? If "look" means 'perceive by hand,' then Kelli should find a way to explore the named object by hand under all these conditions. If "look" means 'perceive, using any modality,' Kelli still *might* seek to explore the objects manually under all conditions, but it is likely that in certain conditions, such as hearing a radio from afar, she might assume she is *already* looking and therefore need do nothing special beyond quieting and orienting to the sound.

In fact, there was no trace of such differential responding under the varying conditions in which the command to "look" was presented. No matter that 'perceive by ear' is a plausible thing to do in response to a radio playing on the other side of the room. When told to "look," in this and all other trials, Kelli retrieved the object and explored it by hand.

Summary comments. Let us now review the results of the first four manipulations. In Experiments 1 and 2 the evidence suggested that *look* meant 'explore by hand' to Kelli. But two responses in Experiment 2 (e.g., the response of sniffing when told to "look with your nose") suggested that *look* might mean 'perceive amodally.' The rarity of this kind of response might represent a bias only. Maybe the hand is usually the best way to explore and apprehend without in principle being the only way, if the command is to "look." Experiments 3 and 4 therefore varied the perceptual command given ("look," "listen," and "taste") or the plausibility of the perceptual modality to the situation (hearable versus haptically explorable situations) in which the command "Look!" was presented. The most straightforward interpretation of the four experiments is that Kelli believes that *look* means 'explore by hand' rather than 'explore by any plausible perceptual means.'

Experiment 5:
How does the sighted child "look with her hands"?

There can be no doubt at all that adults have amodal and cross-modal interpretations of the visual verbs,[2] but we so far have conjectured that the interpretation of *look* for the young sighted child is modality-specific to the eye, as it is specific to the hands for Kelli. Yet it is possible to suppose that the sighted children may be biased toward using their eyes to try to look (accounting for their behavior in Experiment 1, where they oriented the face despite being blindfolded) without in principle denying that they could understand *look* to be interpretable as 'explore haptically,' as it is for Kelli. So it is necessary to ask for the sighted children, as we just did for Kelli, whether the real meaning of *look* is modal or amodal. Therefore we now tried to induce the sighted subjects to behave as Kelli did by asking them specifically to "look with the hands."

Subjects. The four subjects were the same as in Experiments 1 and 2, at the same ages, and again blindfolded.

Stimuli and procedure. The subjects were asked to "look" in different directions just as in Experiment 1, but this time each command called for looking "with your hands," e.g. "Look up with your hands", "Look behind you with your hands", etc., for the six commands given in Experiment 1. The commands were presented in the same order as in Experiment 1.

Results and discussion. The blindfolded children were confused by the request to "look with the hands," even though manual exploration was certainly possible in the situation. In one third of the trials they oriented their heads only, just as in Experiment 1. There was a single trial in which a subject oriented her hands only (without contacting the target object). In the other two thirds of the trials the subjects oriented their heads toward the target object and then tried to do something with their hands as well. But this aspect of their responses was quite odd. For instance, a response to "look up with your hands" was to tilt the head upward (as in Experiment 1, the response to "look up") and simultaneously to position the hands near the face, palms upward, (illustrated in Figure 3.6). Another example of this behavior was a response to "look down with your hands": The subject tilted her head downward and positioned her palms underneath her eyes. That is, the subjects' usual response was to try to mimic visual looking by orienting the head appropriately, and also to do something (quite irrelevant) with their hands. They never were tempted to suppose that the hands could serve as the exploratory organs for looking, despite the specific direction. We conclude that *look* is tied to the visual modality for the sighted children. (For discussion of related findings for blindfolded adults, see note 2 to this chapter).

Discussion

The studies just described were limited to asking about comprehension of the verb *look*, which describes perceptual exploration. Comparable studies were not done for the verb *see*, which describes perceptual states or apprehension. *See* was excluded from these initial studies for reasons that have to do with its sense and

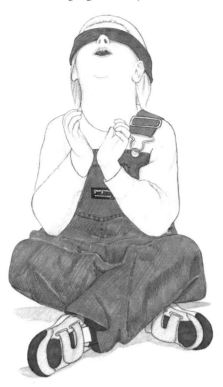

Figure 3.6 *A blindfolded sighted child's response to "look up with your hands." In Experiment 5, the blindfolded children often responded simply by moving their eyes and heads in responses to such commands, but most often moved their eyes and heads and then did something irrelevant with their hands.*

hence the difficulty of obtaining behavioral evidence that a child comprehends this word. Briefly, the problem is that one can hardly command a person to "be in a state of apprehending" and, even if one can, it is hard to tell from that person's subsequent behavior whether he might have *obeyed* the command to "be in a state of apprehending." Nonetheless, Chapter 4 will present limited findings concerning Kelli's distinction between *look* and *see* as these words apply to sighted others. And in Chapter 5 we will give direct evidence from her spontaneous speech that she does understand both *look* and *see* and applies the two terms in different and appropriate circumstances.

Returning now to the studies just presented, it appears that Kelli understood the term *look* to apply to haptic explorations. How is it to be explained that she commandeered the sighted term *look* to encode these haptic explorations? One answer may be social. Perhaps Kelli's parents used the word *look* always and only as they were putting objects into Kelli's hands—and had they instead used *look* when they were rattling objects next to her ear, perhaps she would have thought *look* meant 'listen' instead of 'explore manually.' As we shall show later (Chapters 6 and 7), this social explanation does not survive a close scrutiny of the maternal discourse with Kelli.

Rather, we propose that the basis for Kelli's—and the sighted children's—interpretation turns on the requirement for a term that refers to the dominant mode for the exploration and apprehension of objects. We believe that, to a young child, *look* means 'explore with the dominant modality used for apprehending objects,' distinct from such terms as *touch* that refer merely to manual contact. Neither 'listen' nor 'smell' has this meaning for either population because, as we have stated, these modalities provide only weak inferential evidence as to the nature and existence of objects. We believe that Kelli has achieved the appropriate perceptual-exploratory interpretation of *look*. Her use of the term is tied to the haptic modality because her dominant modality for apprehending objects is manual-kinesthetic. For sighted children of the same age, the use of the same term is tied to the visual modality because that is dominant for them. We would conjecture, similarly, that if some children were sonar-equipped, as bats are, rather than being primarily visual or haptic in their exploratory sensorium, the meaning of *look* would be aural for them.

4 / The Meaning of Sighted Verbs: *Look* and *See* as the Blind Child Applies Them to Others

> He that has not before received into his mind, by the proper inlet, the simple idea which any word stands for, can never come to know the signification of that word by any other words or sounds whatsoever, put together according to any rules of definition. The only way is by applying to his senses the proper object, and so producing that idea in him, for which he has learned the name already.
>
> (John Locke, 1690, Book 3.IV.11)

We have seen that Kelli commandeered the verb *look* to refer appropriately to her own perceptual explorations. But her caregivers seem to live in a partly different perceptual world. Did she assume that they confronted reality the same way she did, that all the world was blind? As we will now show, Kelli construed the sighted terms differently for herself and for sighted people in terms of three properties of vision: Sighted looking and seeing require orientation of the line of sight from eye to object; can be accomplished at a distance; and are blocked by a barrier. Moreover, she seemed to understand the distinction between visual exploratory acts (encoded in English as acts of *looking*) and the resulting states (encoded in English as states of *seeing*). She made this distinction even though she could never perform any visual acts or achieve visual states. Her comprehension implies, perhaps in contradiction to Locke's suggestions as cited above, that learners can acquire lexical items which encode concepts not intimately present to personal perception. Of course we shall not argue from these results that extralinguistic experience plays no role in the acquisition of lexical concepts, even of the concept 'look, as of sighted people,' as understood by a blind child. Indeed, as we will demonstrate, Kelli's learning need not be interpreted as exceeding the bounds of her experience. Rather, her learning dramatizes the requirement for a theory of how the learner organizes experience so as to arrive at coherent lexical representations.

Experiment 1: Orientation of the line of sight

Our first question was whether Kelli knew that sighted persons require orientation of the line of sight in order to see. If so, she should orient an object toward the viewer when asked to "let him or her (visually) see it." To make sure that Kelli discriminated such commands both from "let someone touch it" and from "let someone (manually) see it," we adopted the following general procedure. The object presented for seeing was always out of arm's reach. In addition, a specific side of the object (here, its front or its back) was always mentioned in the command. This was done because that face need not be oriented for tactile exploration of an object: One can move the hand around to the farther side of the object and still touch or manually see it. In contrast, one cannot visually "see around" to the back of objects except with the aid of a periscope.

Stimuli and procedure. At age 42 months, Kelli was asked by the experimenter to "let me see/look at" either "the front of your shirt/pants" or "the back of your shirt/pants," with Kelli either initially facing or facing away from the questioner. Each command was presented while she was standing at a distance between three to five feet from the experimenter so that neither her shirt nor her pants were within *E*'s reach as the command was given. Kelli had access to this distance information because of her ability to localize the sound of the questioner's voice. All combinations of the orienting commands (crossed by *shirt/pants*) yielded eight stimuli, four each front/back and four each initially facing/facing away. As usual, the commands were randomized and presented during play.

Results and discussion. Kelli performed perfectly with 8 out of 8 appropriate orientations (p = .00, Binomial Test). On the trials in which Kelli initially faced *E*, she made no spatial adjustment to let *E* see the front of her (Kelli's) shirt/pants, but simply drew attention to the item by pointing or plucking at it; in contrast, she changed her orientation to let *E* see the back of her pants/shirt. Symmetrically, when she was initially facing away from *E*, she made no adjustment to let *E* see the back of her pants/shirt and

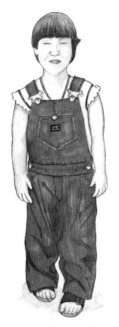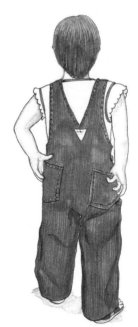

Figure 4.1 *Kelli's response to "let me see the back of your pants. The command is here given while the child is facing the experimenter (1a). Her response is to turn around and pluck at her pants (1b), usually also saying "This the back of my pants." In Experiment 1, the correct orientation was made for each such command.*

turned around to show *E* the front of her shirt/pants (see Figure 4.1 for illustration of these behaviors).

We conclude that Kelli knew that sighted looking requires that the viewer have his front (or face) oriented toward the named face of the object to be seen. Similar evidence on sighted children's sensitivity to the conditions under which viewing can take place has been presented by Flavell and his colleagues (1977; Lempers, Flavell, and Flavell, 1977), though of course the findings for sighted children may be based on default inferences from their own experiences while Kelli's cannot. That is, the sighted learner might implicitly assume something like this: "As my viewing is a function of orientation of my eye to an object, so must the viewing of others be a function of the same variable." Kelli has no simple basis for making such an inference, though as we shall suggest later, it is possible that she makes a related, cross-modal, inference: from her directional haptic explorations to the directional visual explorations of sighted people.

(handwritten margin note: (we assume kellis behavior is less dominant — could be first or vic-versa.)

Experiment 2: Do sighted people see at a distance?

The question here concerns the conditions under which Kelli believed her mother could *see* and *be shown* as against *touch* and *be given* objects that are within reach or are distant. For Kelli herself, it was necessary to come right up to the objects in response to any of these commands, though the particular action—contacting for *touch* and exploring for *see*—would then differ (see Chapter 3). But if Kelli believed that *seeing* and *being shown* can be accomplished at a distance for a sighted observer, she would not necessarily put an object into that observer's hands when presented with such commands.

Stimuli and procedures. At 40 months, Kelli was given sixteen commands, four of each type. She was asked: "Let (either *E* or Mommy) see (an object)," "Let (*E* or Mommy) touch (object)," "Show (*E* or Mommy) (object)," "Give (*E* or Mommy) (object)." The experimenter held Kelli on her lap (the *near* condition), and the mother was positioned three to six feet from Kelli (the *far* condition). Kelli could tell both from the sound of her mother's voice and, directly from being told, that her mother was some distance away. Commands were randomized and presented during play.

Results and discussion. Kelli's responses for the *show/give* and *let see/let touch* distinctions are shown in Table 4.1, row 1, and illustrated in Figures 4.2 and 4.3. She always extended the object toward the target person when asked to *give* or *let touch* (eight of eight trials), but only sometimes (four of eight trials) extended it when asked to *show* or *let see*. This distribution is significant ($p = .038$, Fisher exact test). The fact that she did sometimes give an

Table 4.1 *Do sighted people see at a distance?*

Behavior	Show	Let see	Give	Let touch	Total
I. Experiment 2					
Moves object closer to person	2	2	4	4	12
Does not move object closer to person	2	2	0	0	4
II. Experiment 1					
Moves object closer to person		0			
Does not move object closer to person		8			

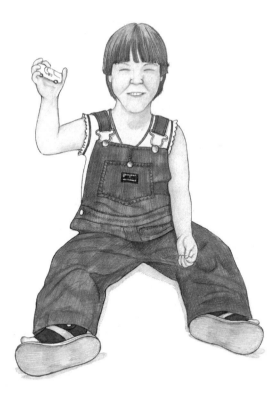

Figure 4.2 *Kelli's response to "let Mommy see the car." In Experiment 2, Kelli responded to commands to let see and show without necessarily moving the object closer to the questioner.*

object to someone when asked to show it is perfectly reasonable—so do you and I, in normal conversational interchange. When anyone is asked to let someone see something, a normal and reasonable tactic is to give it to that person for examination. Hence if a person is asked to "show," we must expect she will sometimes give, i.e., put into the hand. The only question that can therefore be answered by this procedure is whether one *can* be shown at a distance (yes, if one is sighted) and *can* be given at a distance (no, whether blind or sighted). As the table shows, Kelli's responses are consistent with the supposition that she made this distinction.

Though the pattern of responses to *show/let see* versus *give/let touch* are reliably different from each other, the absolute differences are small. But the present interpretation is strengthened by adding the data from Experiment 1 (the orientation probe) to

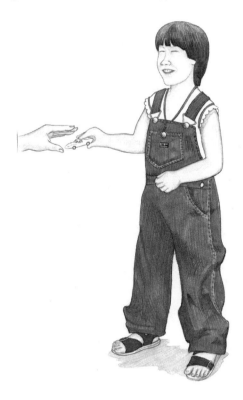

Figure 4.3 *Kelli's response to "let Mommy touch the car." In Experiment 2, Kelli always responded to commands to* let *touch and* give *by moving the object closer to the questioner.*

those so far considered. Recall that in this prior situation Kelli was standing three to five feet from the questioner, who said "Let me see the front/back of your pants/shirt." In this situation the ordinary inference from *let see* to *give* is weakened (it is unlikely that the questioner wants to take your pants to examine them when she says "Let me see the back of your pants"). And so for these commands the item to be seen was never extended toward the questioner. Adding these data (row II of Table 4.1), we can again test for whether the child's tendency to extend the object toward the questioner differs for different verbs; the pattern of responses to *show/let see* versus *give/let touch* are reliably different from each other ($p < .005$, Fisher exact test).

Further supporting evidence for our interpretation comes from additional probes in which we repeatedly urged Kelli to show an object to her father, even though she had already raised the object high—and oriented it toward him—in response to a prior command "Show Daddy." The question was whether she would be easily induced by such misleading conversational circumstances to make the object yet *more* "visible" by putting it into her father's hand. It turned out that Kelli was hard to mislead: Her response in these trying circumstances was to raise the object still higher on each repetition of the command rather than moving it closer to him.

From the behavioral evidence, it is safe to conclude that Kelli believed correctly that sighted looking can take place at a distance, but only if the correct face of the object is positioned in the viewer's line of sight. For completeness, we should add that sometimes Kelli's verbal responses were even more convincing than the behavioral ones. For example, when asked to "let mommy see the doll" she held and shook it close to her own body, saying "I'm just showing her—and it can be in my hand, alright?"

But what if her (in room?)

Experiment 3: Can sighted people see through barriers?

Here we asked whether Kelli knew that barriers prevent seeing by sighted persons, even if the orientation is correct. We tested for this property rather late in Kelli's development (56 months), only because we didn't think to do so sooner. Nothing indicates that Kelli learned about barriers later than about orientations or distances relevant to sighted viewing.

Stimuli and procedure. Kelli was given a randomized set of twelve commands during play. On half of the trials, she was told "Make it so (person) cannot see (object)" and on the other half "Make it so (person) cannot hear (object)." Three objects were used: a Jack-in-the-box, a squeaky fish, and a music box that opened to display a ballerina turning in a circle. Each of these objects gave Kelli the chance to make a noise with or to silence the object, and either to display a part to the viewer or to conceal it.

Results and discussion. The results are illustrated in Figure 4.4. Kelli behaved distinctively and appropriately (twelve out of twelve times) for the three stimulus types ($p = .00$, Binomial Test). When told "Make it so (person) cannot hear (object)," she behaved so as to shut off the sound: She closed the music box (turning it off), took the fish from the person who was squeaking it and held it gingerly by the tail, or stopped winding the Jack. When told "Make it so that (person) cannot see (object)," she actively concealed it from vision. For the Jack, she pushed him down into his cavern; for the ballerina, she either closed the box or covered it

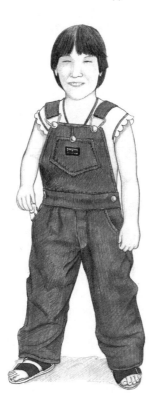

Figure 4.4 *Kelli's response to "make it so Mommy cannot see the car." She hides it in her pocket. In Experiment 3, Kelli concealed objects from view in response to the command "make it so I cannot see X," and silenced objects in response to "make it so I cannot hear X."*

with her hand, saying "She's sleeping"; for the fish, she tried to fit it into the music box or Jack box and close the lid. When this attempt failed with the Jack box because it was too small, she said "I'm gonna put it under the chair," which she did, adding "Now she can't see it."

Spontaneous observations accord with those in these elicited situations. For example, one day Kelli jumped into her bed, drew the covers over her, and cried out "Anybody can't see me now!" Notice that the cloth would be a barrier to sight and not to haptic exploration, for one can feel but not see through the material, suggesting that Kelli's knowledge may have been quite refined before age five.

We conclude that Kelli knew about a number of kinds of barrier that can prevent a sighted person from seeing, even when the distance and orientation of the objects were correct for sighted seeing.

Experiment 4: Seeing with the eye and with the hand

We began discussion in this chapter by asking whether Kelli distinguished between the way she herself sees and the way sighted individuals see. We have so far demonstrated that she responded differently to commands having to do with vision (*see* of others) and commands having to do with haptic exploration (*see* of a blind person). A further question was whether she realized that, for sighted people, it matters which organ is used exploratorily: The eye sees in one way, the hand sees in another. Did Kelli even know that her mother could explore manually (and constrained by such properties of the haptic sensorium as the requirement for physical contact) even though she could explore visually as well (i.e., at a distance, etc.)?

Materials and procedure. This issue was investigated when Kelli was 56 months old.[1] She was given a set of sixteen commands that specifically named the organ her mother was to use: Half of them were "Let Mommy see with her eyes," and the other half were "Let Mommy see with her hands." Half of the command types were given far from the mother (at least five feet) and half were given close to her (within arm's reach). Half were given with large objects, such as an 18-inch-long doll, and half with very small objects such as one-half-inch-long Lego parts. The commands were randomized and presented during play.

Results. Table 4.2 presents the results for the eye/hand distinc-

Table 4.2 *Experiment 4: Seeing with the eye and with the hand*

Command and object position	Moves object closer	Does not move object closer
Let Mommy see with her eyes		
Near	2[a]	2
Far	0	4
Let Mommy see with her hands		
Near	4	0
Far	4	0

a. In both of these commands, Kelli extended the object slightly towards the mother.

tion. In all eight cases of "Let mommy see with her hands" Kelli either placed the object in her mother's hands or demanded that her mother "come over" or "come here," and then she placed the object in her mother's hands. This was done no matter whether the objects were quite close to the mother to start with or were relatively distant. In clear contrast, none of the "Let mommy see with her eyes" commands induced Kelli to place the object in her mother's grasp. In two of the eight instances of this type, she did extend the object toward the mother, though not all the way to her; in the remaining six instances, she held the object up to view, moving it no closer to the mother. This pattern of results is statistically significant (p = .034, Fisher exact test). Again, the near/far distinction was immaterial to the response style. It is reasonable to conclude that Kelli believed her mother capable of both manual and visual exploration; it also is reasonable to conclude that Kelli knew that the conditions for these two kinds of exploration differ systematically.

Further findings of interest from this probe had to do with Kelli's manner of displaying large and small objects for visual inspection (for the eight commands "Let mommy see with her eyes"). As just stated, Kelli held the object up or out for viewing and turned it toward her mother in each such command. Further, her hand shape—how she held the object so it could be inspected—differed according to the size of the object. For the small Lego pieces, she displayed them on her open palm. For large objects, she would simply grasp them and dangle them. The point here is that Kelli behaved as though she knew that if her hand closed around a very small object, this created a barrier to visual inspection (see again Experiment 3), whereas closure of the hand around some small part of a large object did not prevent visual inspection (of most of that object).

As so often, Kelli's verbal responses sometimes give even clearer evidence of her knowledge of such facts than do the behavioral responses. When told "Let mommy see the Lego with her eyes," Kelli displayed the object on the open palm but also cautioned "Alright, but it's gonna fall out!" In short, she knew that the open hand was required if her mother was to see the object visually—but the consequence would be an insecure grasp.

Experiment 5: Does the blind child differentiate between active and stative visual verbs?

None of the probes reported so far require us to believe that Kelli could differentiate one sighted verb from another. As mentioned briefly in Chapter 3, *look* and *see*, though semantically related, differ in meaning in interesting ways. One distinction has to do with the fact that the primary use of *look* is to encode acts of exploration, while *see* is primarily used to encode the resultant mental state. To understand this distinction, notice that there is a non-contradictory reading of "I must have looked at that a dozen times, but I never saw it." That is to say, one can engage in a perceptual activity (exploring with the eye or with the hand) without arriving at the mental state that is ordinarily its consequence (perceiving visually or haptically).[2]

We now asked whether Kelli differentiated active *look* and stative *see*, as these apply to events involving sighted people. As a control for whether Kelli made the active/stative distinction at all (when using verbs that encode it for her intact sensoria), she was also tested for the same distinction as it is made in the auditory mode and encoded in the active term *listen* versus the stative term *hear*.

Method and results.[3] At age 54 months, Kelli was told "We're going to fool Mommy. We're going to tell her to look (at a Jack that can pop out of a box) but then we won't let the Jack pop." Similarly, she was told "We're going to tell her to listen (to a squeaky toy) but then we won't squeak it." Kelli performed these acts (two trials of each) without difficulty. She said to her mother "Look!" and then did not pop the Jack. The experimenter then asked Kelli "Did Mommy look?" Kelli replied "Yes." And "Did Mommy see?" Kelli replied, "No." When asked why, she responded on one trial "The Jack didn't pop," and on the other, "We fooled her." The same result was achieved for the auditory verbs: When asked "Did Mommy listen?" she responded "Yes," but to "Did Mommy hear?" she responded "No" and gave the same kind of justification, "We didn't squeak it."

Ideally, this manipulation should have been replicated with more trials and more stimulus objects. But the game quickly palled for both Kelli and her mother. We shall present supportive evidence in Chapter 5, where the same distinctions are shown to be made in Kelli's spontaneous speech. But the present data already suggest that Kelli could make at least some of the distinctions between *look* and *see* (for sighted others) that we would expect for a sighted language learner of similar age and that she is in a position to make for the auditory-perceptual verbs.

What Visual Terms Mean to Their Users

In Chapter 3, we showed that Kelli construed *look* as describing her own haptic explorations. In the present chapter, we have shown that Kelli understood *look/see* and *show/give* differently as these words apply to sighted individuals, in terms of the major properties that distinguish vision from haptic exploration. Sighted seeing can be at a distance, requires orientation of the line of sight, and is blocked even by barriers through which the hand can extract information (such as a soft cloth). Moreover, sighted vision involves active visual exploration (*looking*), which may or may not lead to visual perception (*seeing*).

How are these findings to be described? We have concluded that *look,* as used by any learner—blind or sighted—means 'explore objects by use of the dominant modality.' Thus for all the children, we claimed that the construal was tied to a modality, not amodal. The only difference between Kelli and sighted children was the modality that *look* identified: the eye for sighted children, the hand for blind children. This claim was based primarily on the following findings: (1) In responding to "look at," say, a distant playing radio, Kelli should sometimes merely have quieted and oriented her ear because listening would be the most obvious way of perceiving under these conditions, but she did not (as demonstrated in Experiments 3 and 4 of Chapter 3). Thus listening does not seem to be an acceptable instance of *looking,* though surely it is an instance of perceiving. This suggests that *look* cannot simply mean 'perceive.' (2) The blindfolded sighted children should have had a natural interpretation for "look with your hands" when their eyes were covered, if they believed that *look* meant 'amodally perceive'; they should have explored by use of their hands, but they did not (as demonstrated in Experiment 5 of Chapter 3). This suggests that to them looking requires vision in particular.

We have also demonstrated that Kelli understands *look* and *see* as used of sighted individuals in a way that is responsive to the different spatial perceptions and inferences available to the eye and the hand. Again, this result is best interpreted by assuming that Kelli interprets the visual terms as modality tied—though now two different modalities are implicated, depending on the sensorium of the user. This conclusion is based primarily on two main findings from the present chapter: (1) Kelli was able to comprehend that perception could take place both by hand and by eye for sighted people (Experiment 4, this chapter). So (2) in responding to *show/let see* versus *give/let touch* of sighted others, she should have been equally likely to put objects in their hands for any of these commands, if she believed that these words encoded all and any forms of perception—but she was not (Experiments 1 and 2).

We conclude that the modal interpretation of visual verbs is more revealing of the comprehension performances of Kelli and the sighted blindfolded subjects as well (though, to be sure, adults seem comfortable enough with cross-modal and amodal interpretations of the same words). Kelli was different from the sighted children in only one important way. She seemed to assume that *looking* and *seeing* might be performed in different ways, that her mother could see either with her hands or with her eyes.[4]

Summarizing, the most straightforward interpretation of all these results, taken together, is that Kelli formed two lexical entries for each sight-related verb, one applicable to visual viewing only—never to Kelli's own acts and explorations—and the other applicable to manual viewing—the only mode for Kelli herself and applicable to sighted seeing only if specially marked ('see with the hands'). Thus Kelli was able to construe *look* and *see* in one way ('explore by hand') that derives rather transparently from aspects of her own exploratory sensorium. But, at the same time, she was able to construe *look* and *see* in another way ('explore by eye'), one that is remote from her own interactions with the world of objects, scenes, and events.

The findings for the *look/see* distinction (Experiment 5) make similar points. Kelli could neither look nor see by visual means; she could not apprehend in any direct way how others can do this. How then could she, even less securely, infer a distinction *between* these two terms as they apply to sighted people: that one is active and the other stative? Yet evidently she has accomplished enough learning to know that there are occasions on which her mother looked but did not see.

Learning and Experience: More Questions

These findings return us to the debate on how extralinguistic experience is used to learn the meaning of words. At first glance our results might suggest—*pace* Locke—that learners can acquire information about lexical items without guidance from external experience. Kelli did learn much about visual viewing (as her sighted sister learned something about blind viewing, see note 4). But such a conclusion would be extravagant. The findings so far presented really pose no principled difficulty for a context-driven theory of lexical concept attainment, surprising as this may seem.

Kelli's experience does provide haptic analogies to the spatial properties of visual *look/see*. The ears, like the eyes, are distance receptors; barriers sometimes (though not always) block haptic exploration much as they block visual exploration; and haptic exploration is directional, as is visual exploration. It is these spatial properties of visual seeing that Kelli came to know about. If she made just these analogies from her own perceptual world to account for what others seem to know, her knowledge of sighted *see* is probably explained. Similarly, Kelli has direct experience in the auditory mode (listening versus hearing) as well as the tactile mode (touching versus feeling) relevant to the active/stative distinction among verbs. Hence her acquisition of this distinction for the visual mode of others may well have been dependent on these available experiential bases, which made a cross-modal analogy available to her. In short, Kelli's experiential inductive base does provide information that could be relevant in some way to her construction of the concept of visual viewing.

There is evidently a rich experiential basis for Kelli's inductions. But acknowledging this goes almost no distance in explaining these inductions. Once we have asserted that Kelli "learned from experience," it remains as mysterious as ever just how she used experience in exactly the right ways to arrive at the correct construals of the terms we have investigated. The real task in understanding her language learning is to work out how she learned from experience in a way that will predict only the correct analogies to vision—as opposed to a variety of other conjectures and analogies that experience could have made available. As one example, she might have assumed that her mother meant 'hope to or try to apprehend (manually)' by *see*; this would have accounted just as well for why the mother was willing to say "I see" when she was at a distance from relevant objects.

Summarizing, we part company with those investigators of language learning who proclaim that this feat is explained in terms of the availability of extralinguistic experience. What we do not doubt is that Kelli's experience was rich enough to provide a basis for building the visual construals of visual terms, as these describe the perceptions and explorations of others as well as herself. What we do doubt is that a general theory of induction can predict that Kelli's extralinguistic experiences necessarily conspire to yield exactly these lexical concepts and no others. Who told Kelli that, to understand *look/see* properly, the appropriate aspects of experience to recruit in evidence are those relevant to a spatial geometry relating sighted individuals to objects when they say of those objects "I see"? The real problem in understanding the attainment of lexical concepts is to identify the particular properties and organizations of experience that are selected by the learner, to explain how the induction of word meaning is so constrained that only the correct analogies are drawn. To this question, the answer that "there is extralinguistic experience" is insufficient.

5 / Saying *Look* and *See*, and Judging How to Do So

Information about Kelli's construal of the visual verbs has so far come from comprehension performances. Two more evidentiary sources are now discussed: Kelli's spontaneous productions and her "metalinguistic" or judgmental performance with these verbs.

The child's spontaneous production of the visual verbs is important for two reasons. First, it has frequently been suggested that production and comprehension may differ from each other more in young children than in adults (e.g., Bever, 1970; Goldin-Meadow, Seligman, and Gelman, 1976). Therefore we cannot simply assume that Kelli's ability to understand *look* and *see* when appropriately used by others implies that she can produce the words appropriately herself; rather it is necessary to demonstrate the extent to which this is so. Second, the production data from Kelli give us particularly clear information about her distinction between active *look* and stative *see*, an issue for which the comprehension data presented so far are quite limited (to the few probes in Experiment 5 of Chapter 4).

Kelli's judgments as to the conditions for blind and sighted *looking* and *seeing* are also presented. These were collected when she was six years old, for while even two-year-olds can talk and understand, it is quite difficult to get preschoolers to comment explicitly about language and its use. These late-appearing metalinguistic performances are of some interest for they give some idea of how far the blind child might be able to go in her understanding of sighted looking and seeing and the terms that encode them. The comprehension and production data are of course the more basic, and tell us about language knowledge in the sense that the user knows when and how to apply a word to external events. The judgmental data add information pertaining to how explicit and conscious this knowledge may eventually become. Young children are notoriously limited in their ability to give language judgments—or, for that matter, almost any kind of judgment—on demand (cf. Gleitman, Gleitman, and Shipley, 1972; DeVilliers and DeVilliers, 1972; Hirsch-Pasek, Gleitman, and Gleitman, 1978). Therefore we will also describe findings from blind and deaf-blind adults whose explicit knowledge of visual terminology (as tested by asking them for definitions) goes well beyond that of Kelli at six years of age.

Spontaneous Production

All of Kelli's spontaneous uses of *look* and *see* (190 instances) that occurred during the videotaped sessions from ages 30–60 months (twenty-one sessions, averaging one hour in length) were culled from the tapes and coded in various ways. An attempt was also made to determine if they were used appositely to the real-world circumstances in which they were uttered.

Syntactic formats

Table 5.1 shows Kelli's use of *look* and *see*. In 59 percent of the cases, they occurred in simple transitive sentences followed by a noun-phrase (NP) object. Not surprisingly, the complexity of these sentences (and indeed of all syntactic types) changed with age. Thus at 30 months Kelli said "See camera!"; at 37 months, "I'm gonna see Miss Barbara"; at 40 months, "I gonna come over see Tabatha"; and by 55 months, "Here, you can see the other bottle too, Sommer." In a further 11 percent of the cases, *look* and *see* were used intransitively, e.g., "I can't see." Simple (one-word) deictic interjectives ("Look!" or "See?") accounted for another 21 percent of the cases. Seven percent more consisted of interjectives followed immediately—and intonationally within the same sentence contour—by a deictic sentence, e.g., "See? It's in my lap" (36 months), or "Look, I got Legos" (39 months). In the remaining 2 percent of the cases, *see* occurred with simple sentential complements, e.g., "See the camera be on" (meaning something like "I want to see how the camera is on," said after we discussed among ourselves the question of whether the camera was on, 35 months); and *look* occurred with free relatives such as *what* or *how* (e.g., "Look what I have!" or "Look how I do it!," uttered at 36 months). One time only, Kelli used *look like* in the sense of 'resemble' ("You look like Daddy").

Table 5.1 *Frequencies of Kelli's spontaneous uses of* look *and* see

Syntactic formats	Questions SP[a]	Questions PP[b]	Imperatives SP	Imperatives PP	Declaratives SP	Declaratives PP	Totals SP	Totals PP
See + NP	14	6	2	–	46	3	62	9
Look at NP	–	–	33	–	3	5	36	5
Look!	–	–	24	–	2	–	26	–
See?	12	–	–	–	–	–	12	–
See? + S (deictic)	6	–	–	–	1	–	7	–
Look! + S (deictic)	–	–	5	–	–	–	5	–
See? + S (other)	2	–	–	–	1	–	3	–
Look! + S (other)	–	–	1	–	–	–	–	–
Look + NP	–	–	–	–	–	2	–	2
See (intransitive)	1	–	–	–	19	–	20	–
Look (intransitive)	–	–	–	–	1	–	1	–
Look like	–	–	–	–	1	–	1	–

Note: This table represents only those formats actually occurring in Kelli's speech. There are in principle many other formats that could have occurred, but did not. Two such formats that merit special mention are queries using *look* (e.g., Look?) and imperatives using *see* (e.g., See!).
a. Simple present.
b. Present progressive.

Appropriateness of use

The utterances were examined for their appositeness to ongoing scenes and events. But on this topic there is very little detail that can be extracted from watching the scene. Indeed, we never observed a use of *look* or *see* that seemed bizarre. As we remarked earlier, it is not so obvious that one could tell if some spontaneous usage really *was* bizarre, appearances aside. For one thing, the relations between real-world events and speech events is indirect at best (just the problem that language learners must confront, but also and for the same reasons just the problem that investigators of children's language must confront). These interpretive problems are exacerbated for verbs of the kind we are studying. Since *look* and *see* encode the speaker's exploratory perceptions (which are invisible) and mental states (which are even more invisible), they can be uttered in almost any imaginable state of affairs in the world: Their appropriateness depends on how the user is representing the outside world and his exploration of it to himself at the moment; of this we can have no sure knowledge. Nonetheless, the production data, as compared against their real-world contexts, do show that Kelli's use of *see* and *look at* was appropriate, and in line with the comprehension data presented in Chapters 3 and 4; and that she distinguished between *look* and *see* in her speech in ways that are normal for children of her age.

The exploration of objects and events

Almost all noninterjective uses of *see* and *look at*, as interpreted against the context of use, seemed best construed as comments, requests, and commands to explore an object. Only very occasionally did the construal 'contact' seem as natural, but this usage is very clear in two early productions, when Kelli (37 months) said "Don't see that, Sommer!" and then "Sommer, don't see that," pushing her sister's hand away from Kelli's record player. Only once did the word *touch* appear in the corpus of utterances, as a comment on the mother's activity: "You're looking at it and touching it" (44 months). A few utterances of *look* and *see* also or alternatively expressed the location or direction of the exploration, e.g., "I'm looking out the window," said while Kelli was facing a window. A few uses concerned exploration of an object as embedded in an event (e.g., "Look, I have a bag of beads" or "Look what I have," said while holding up a bag of beads). Overall, then, Kelli spontaneously uttered *look* and *see* in circumstances that seem to accord with the ways she comprehended them, namely to describe the exploration of objects and the location and directions of those explorations, in which cases the verb was followed by an NP object; and to refer to exploration and apprehension of an event or state of affairs, in which case a descriptive sentence was adjoined to *look* with a free relative (such as *how*) or occurred as the complement of *see*.

The active/stative distinction

Despite Kelli's experiential deprivations, her spontaneous speech makes clear that she honored a crucial linquistic and conceptual distinction between *look* and *see*. This is the distinction mentioned for Experiment 5 of Chapter 4, between active *look* and stative *see*. This experiment suggested that Kelli knew of circumstances when her mother might actively explore visually (*look*) or auditorily (*listen*) but still not perceive or apprehend (*see* or *hear*).

Interjective commands. The clearest syntactic format which suggests that Kelli made the active/stative distinction in her own speech is the single-word interjective. Notice that in Table 5.1 there are *no* single-word interjective instances in which Kelli said "Look?" (tried to use *look* as an interjective query) or said "See!"

(tried to use *see* as an interjective command or request). These choices are fully in accord with the same distinction as made by adults. The absence of the imperative *See!* format and the presence of the imperative *Look!* format are explainable on semantic grounds. As we stated in Chapter 4, it is conceptually coherent to command someone to look, i.e., to perform an act, but it is less coherent to command someone to see, i.e., to be in a particular mental state. (That would be thought control.) Hence stative verbs in English often sound very odd in command contexts: "Suspect Mary of treason!" or "Think John has left!" or "See the dog!" This prohibition is not really categorical ("See the dog!" is awkward, or perhaps takes on a vocative interpretation such as "Lo, the dog!" but does not seem impossible). But the restriction is very strong in the interjective, single-word, context in particular: *"See!" (meaning "I command you to see!") sounds unnatural. Accordingly, Kelli never says this. In contrast, active verbs sound fine in these environments: "Accuse Mary of treason!", "Make sure that John has left!", "Look at the dog!" and "Look!". Accordingly, we find that Kelli spontaneously said "Look!" when she seemed to want another person to explore or attend to some object or event.

As for commands longer than a single word, these prohibitions, though weaker, still obtain. There are only two instances (and these appear early in development) where Kelli uses *see* commands ("Don't see that, Sommer!" and "Sommer, don't see that!"). In contrast, there are 63 instances of Kelli using *look* commands (e.g., "Look what I have," and "Here Scooter, look at the harmonica!").

Look and see in queries. There are corresponding conceptual (and hence syntactic) restrictions on active *look* and stative *see* in queries, but the syntactic manifestations of these in English are somewhat more complex than for the case of commands. Conceptually it is coherent to ask both whether a person is performing an activity (looking) and whether he is in some mental state (seeing). But clearly there is a complication here, for one can say "See?" while "Look?" sounds very odd, though we have just argued that it is conceptually sensible. The oddity of "Look?" derives from yet another syntactic reflex of the active/stative distinction: Active verbs, when used to express an action taking place in present time, commonly occur in the present progressive rather than the simple present tense, and necessarily so in queries ("Are you eating dinner?" or "Are you looking at the moon?"). This is not to say that the simple present is ungrammatical or unacceptable with such verbs; rather, the construal changes. In such formats, active verbs refer to a timeless, habitual, or generic description of events.

"Do you eat dinner?" is likely a query about someone's long-term dining habits; "Do you look at the moon?" is likely a query about the professional specialty of an astronomer.

In direct contrast, the stative verbs require the simple present and sound distinctly odd with the present progressive. "Are you owning a Picasso?" and "Are you seeing the moon?" sound odder than "Do you own a Picasso?" or "Do you see the moon?" Symmetrically, used to refer to an ongoing, habitual, or repetitive activity rather than to refer to the present moment, the oddity goes away: It is natural to say "Are you seeing an analyst?"

These generalizations in hand, we can return to the question of why speakers, including Kelli, do not say "Look?" The answer is that *look*, an active verb, requires this progressive, and so one must say "Are you looking?" or, much more rarely, "Looking?" The absence of "Look?" does not turn on the conceptual unnaturalness of asking someone if he is currently exploring something. It turns on a further, more subtle, syntactic reflex of the active/stative distinction: the preference for the progressive with active verbs and the preference for the simple present with stative verbs.

For queries longer than the one-word interjective, Kelli's performance breaks down. As has been documented elsewhere (Gleitman et al., 1972), children of Kelli's age do not observe the constraint against progressive *see* in queries very well, hardly surprising given the complexity of this feature of English. Kelli correctly used the simple present for queries containing *see* 80 percent of the time (twenty-three instances, e.g., "See?, it has lid on it," and "See my bed?") but there are quite a few violations (six instances, e.g., "Are you seeing it?" and "Mommy, are you seeing it?").

Summary

We have shown that Kelli predominantly used the visual verbs to describe exploration rather than simple contact with objects and events; and that, overwhelmingly, she used them in ways that honor the active/stative distinction. Thus her spontaneous utterance of visual verbs was systematic in the meanings conveyed and in their appropriateness to the scenes and events around her, and generally in agreement with the syntactic choices standardly made by the linguistic community for the expression of perceptual activities and states. Thus evidence from both speech and comprehension supports the idea that a blind child can learn the meanings of *look* and *see*.

Elicited Descriptions of Meanings

For the period of time through six years, there was little evidence that Kelli had explicit knowledge of her special sensory limitation. All the evidence we have presented pertains to implicit knowledge about visual seeing. For completeness, when Kelli was six, we queried her about her own and others' seeing, to see if her commentary about looking and seeing was in accord with her comprehension and production of these words.

Does sighted seeing require line of sight orientation?

B: What would happen if someone was very far away and they were walking toward us?
K: We could see them.
B: When could we see them?
K: When they were in front.
B: How about if we're standing with our backs to you?
K: You can't see.
B: How come?
K: Because your eyes are facing this way (*points opposite way*).

Can sighted seeing occur at a distance?

B: Could we see something with our eyes up in the sky?
K: I can't because my eyes don't work.
B: Could you touch something up in the sky?
K: No because it is way up here (*reaches her arms up*).
B: How about me? Could I see something up in the sky?
K: Yeah.

What are the organs of sight?

B: How do we see? What do we see with?
K: You guys see with your eyes.
B: And how about you?
K: No.
B: No?
K: I see with my hands

Does light affect visual or haptic seeing?

B: What happens when we turn off the lights?
K: We can't see.
B: Who can't see?
K: Me and you and Mommy and Kathy.
B: How come you can't all see if the lights go off?
K: I don't know.
B: OK, when we turn out the light can you see things with your hands?
K: Yeah.

B: When we turn out the light can we see things with our eyes?
K: No.
. . .

B: Can Mommy see with her eyes when she's outside in the daylight?
K: No.
B: She cannot see, outside in the daytime with her eyes?
K: No, because they're closed like this (*closes her eyes*).
B: How about if they're open?
K: She can see then.
B: Can Mommy see with her eyes when she's outside and it's night-
   time?
K: No.
B: How come?
K: Because it's dark.

Do the eyes have to be open for seeing to occur?

B: Can I see you if my eyes are open?
K: Yes.
B: How come?
K: Because your eyes work.
B: How about if I close my eyes?
K: You can't.
B: How come?
K: Because your eyes are shut.

Is vision blocked by a barrier?

B: How about if the door is closed and I'm standing inside the room
   with you, can I see you then?
K: Yes.
B: Can we see people through a window?
K: My eyes don't work.
B: Could you feel someone through a window? With your hands?
K: No, because they are way outside.
B: How about if there was a big thick curtain in front of the window,
   could we see someone then?
K: No.
B: How come?
K: Because.

Clearly, Kelli has some beginning conscious knowledge of the
differing properties of blind and sighted seeing. But this knowledge is by no means complete, fully correct, or stable, as the following interchanges show:

B: How about if I cover up *your* eyes? (*puts hands over K's eyes*)
K: Like a blindfold?
B: What is a blindfold?
K: Covers up your eyes.
B: What happens if you cover up your eyes?

K: You can't see.
B: Who can't?
K: I can't.
B: How about if I cover up *my* eyes?
K: You can't see.
B: How about if I covered up just one eye?
K: You can't see. If you open your mouth you can.
B: What do you mean?
K: We can't see with our mouth?
B: How come?
K: Because if there's food in it we can see.

Notice that Kelli is easily confused: She doesn't know that one eye can work if the other is covered, and if she is pushed too hard, she begins to wander toward odd inferences about the mouth doing service for the covered eye. One more incident makes this point clearer. Sommer (the younger sister) was observed holding an orange in front of her own eyes, chanting "You can't see my eyesie-eyesie-eyesies!" Kelli proceeded to grab the orange, moving it to various positions in front of her (Kelli's) eyes, apparently trying to figure out what this could mean. Shortly thereafter, B questioned Kelli further about vision:

B: OK. If you're inside at nighttime and there's no light on, can you see with your eyes?
K: No.
B: No . . . How come?
K: 'Cause there's two hands on my orange.
B: Because there's two hands on your orange?
K: Um, two of *my* hands.
B: Two of your hands on your orange, that's why you can't see it inside at night?
K: Right.
B: No—you're being silly. Why can't you see inside at night?
K: Because the light is off.

Kelli clearly has some conscious knowledge of sighted seeing, but it is limited, fragile (subject to collapse if the question is hard) and sometimes downright incorrect. This is all the more surprising because the implicit knowledge that allows Kelli to behave systematically in response to requests and commands that involve the seeing of others is so stable and refined.

The distinction between what is known implicitly, and thus describes behavior, and what can be elicited in reflective tasks, is shown even more dramatically by Kelli's sister's responses in the same kind of task. Recall (note 4, Chapter 4) that Sommer by the age of four was behaviorally accommodating to Kelli's blindness, bringing an object right up to Kelli whether asked to *give, show, let touch,* or *let see.* Nevertheless, at five years old, despite continuous experience with a blind child, Sommer responded to questions not much more insightfully than the blindfolded sighted three-year-olds of Chapter 3:

B: How does Kelli look up?
S: Like this (*tilts her head up*).
B: How does Kelli look down?
S: (*tilts her head down*).
B: How does Kelli look behind her?
S: Like that (*turns her head to look behind*).
B: (*giving hints now*) How does Kelli look up, with her eyes or with her hands?
S: With her eyes (*looks up*).
B: I have the doll in front of you. If you're Kelli, how would Kelli look at the doll?
S: I don't know because I can't see.
B: How would Kelli look at it?
S: She'd go like this (*takes doll in her arms*).
B: With her hands or with her eyes would she look at it?
S: With her hands.

Here the spontaneous bias of the child is to believe that *look* and *see* have to do with vision, so if Kelli is going to look, she'd have to use her eyes; only the series of leading questions extracts any acknowledgment that Kelli looks with the hands. It seems that Kelli and Sommer are limited (though not completely incompetent) in their ability to reflect consciously on the sensory capabilities of others, despite extensive experience. This limit on explicit knowledge contrasts dramatically with their behavioral accommodations to other people, which is extensive and stable.

Definitions from Blind Adults

A question remains whether the blind ever become able to discourse about sighted terms in a way that would lead us to believe they have acquired explicit knowledge of this semantic field despite their own sensory deprivations. The answer here is clearly positive. To see this point, we now report extracts from the same kind of interview, conducted with an adult (twenty years old) who has been blind since birth. Of course, it is always possible to suppose that what a blind adult knows about these matters is the result of explicit and conscious tutoring, in which case it would not be of much interest to the issue of natural language learning. However—particularly for this individual's definitions of sighted terms—it seems unlikely that she was specifically and formally taught each of them.

Characteristics of sighted seeing

Here, a blind adult (D) answers questions concerning the conditions under which sighted seeing could occur.

B: If there was a closed door and I was sitting on one side and you were sitting on the other side of the door, would I be able to see you?

D: If the door had no glass in it you wouldn't.

B: What if we were standing ten feet from each other and there is no intervening barrier?

B: Yes.

B: We're one city block from each other.

D: If it is a clear day and there's nothing . . . I think so; I can't remember how far it is that you can't.

B: What if I'm standing so that we are touching back to back?

D: No. 'Cause you're facing in the opposite direction that I am and you're looking in the opposite direction.

B: What if I'm sitting as I am now across from you and I have my head 90 degrees to the side?

D: Yes, out of the corners of your eyes.

B: Sitting face to face, what if I had my head further than 90 degrees?

D: Maybe a little bit but not too much.

B: Which way would my eyes be pointing . . . Does that make sense to you, to have one's eyes point?

D: Oh yeah, you have to see by having your eyes look directly at something. That's the difference between seeing and hearing. You have to be in the direct line of the object. You can't see all around like you can hear all around.

B: Which way would my eyes be pointing if I was going to look at you and I was standing on a chair and I was looking at you?

D: Depends on if you're a tall or a short person.

B: OK, I'm a tall person.

D: OK, you'd probably have to point them down.

Definitions of sighted words

The same blind adult provides definitions of sighted terms that we think compare well with those one might expect from any intelligent sighted individual.

to look: To see. To use your eyes to perceive something, to get an image of it, to know it's there.

the difference between look and see: You look with your eyes, and how you see is how you interpret it. It's like *hear* and *listen,* you hear the sounds and when you interpret them is when you listen [note that the subject is correct about *look/see*, but has *hear/listen* backwards].

to notice: To see something that comes into your view. But not only to see it but to perceive it and understand it. You could sit on this rocking chair and not notice the color of it at all. Might have to be looking at something specifically to notice it.

to blur: To be unclear, to make you not able to see from a glare.

to conceal: To hide, to block from somebody's view, by putting something in front of it or in back of it in the line of vision.

to darken: To make it dark, or else to add more of a dark color, to add more black.

to dazzle: To brighten, to make it so bright that you can't see for a second, something sudden . . . like turning on a bright light in a dark room. But also isn't it more like shimmering, glowing? Like you think of it with jewels.

to examine: To look at, to scrutinize, to look at it in very fine detail. [E: How do people do that? Would you hold it close to you?] It depends on the size of the object you're looking at. What kind of perspective you want to get on it. If you wanted to get the full detail you would close . . . if you wanted to see a lot of detail you would look at it from far away. If you wanted to see just part of it you would look at it up close.

to expose: to light, like film. To uncover to make something plain. To show something hidden that was not known.

to fade: To disappear gradually . . . sound or color would become less intense, become washed away so the color looks lighter. . . an object will fade as you get further back from it.

to gaze: To look at something intensely. An equivalent would be to listen to something very hard.

to glance: To look at something quickly.

to glare: To look at something weirdly as if you're mad at them.

to obscure: To hide it well, to make it disappear from vision, but it is different from *conceal* 'cause it has it darken. Like leaves obscuring the sign.

to overlook: Not to look over. To miss. To not notice.

to peek: Little kids . . . peek out from over a blanket. Give a quick little look and then go hide again.

Evidently, much can be acquired by the blind about the properties of visual perception and about the rich and specific ways these properties are encoded in a natural language. Perhaps most dramatically of all, C. Chomsky (1984) has investigated definitions of sighted terms by adults who are both deaf and blind. These individuals, deprived of hearing and sight since infancy, acquired language by touch (by placing a hand on the face and neck of the speaker, a method known as Tadoma) and then learned to speak through long years of articulatory training. Definitions of

sighted terms from one of Chomsky's subjects are fully comparable to those provided by the blind adult we just described:

> *stare:* Stare? Well, stare means to stare at a person or an object, maybe
> in surprise or maybe spellbound. For instance, when somebody says
> something to you and you are shocked at what you heard, you stare
> at the person as if you are asking a person a question, because you
> can't believe what he just said. Or to stare, because you are concen-
> trating more deeply into an object. So, you will stare at it, trying to
> focus your mind on what you are looking at.
>
> *dazzle:* When there's a beautiful burst of colors coming at you, you get
> dazzled. Or you get dazzled by a strong burst of light.
>
> *glare:* Glare? Oh, I see, dazzle and glare. Well, when the TV lights glare
> at you, then you get dazzled from the glare. Or if a person is very
> angry at you, he would glare at you. That means almost like stare,
> but glare. Glare means almost like staring at you but he's angry.
> When a person is offended he will glare at you from behind.

A Prospectus for Explanation

It seems clear enough from the findings presented in the last three
chapters that to say language is learned from extralinguistic context does not say enough. A blind child does understand and produce apparently visual terms acquired from a context that is quite
different from that of the sighted learner. And blind—even deaf
and blind—adults can *define* a variety of words that have to do
with the visible world and visual experience. Obviously their information did not come from looking around or looking at others
who were looking around. Since the extralinguistic cues seem to
be inadequate to describe the learning, at least some of the information must have come from elsewhere. There evidently is one
further rich source of information that these individuals could
have used. This is the information that exists in the linguistic environment itself, the organized forms of sentences in which the
visual words figure. We therefore now turn to the question of
what Kelli's linguistic and extralinguistic circumstances for learning really were like.

6 / How Kelli
Learned Visual Terms:
The Environmental Model

Now that it has been determined what Kelli knows about the visual verbs, we arrive at the third question posed in Chapter 1: How does the blind learner acquire these meanings? Obviously there was something in Kelli's environment that provided the evidentiary basis for what she learned. Part of the solution may well lie in the extralinguistic contexts in which she encountered various verbs, including *look* and *see*. For there are probably some reasonably systematic situational concomitants for the use of each verb that language users honor. For example, it would surely be odd to say to a listener "Pick up the ball" or "Take off your clothes" if the listener was already holding the ball and was naked to boot.

To approach this topic of apposite conversational uses of verbs, we examined the natural circumstances in which Kelli's mother uttered common verbs to the child. As we will show, extralinguistic information in the conversational settings does seem to account for part of what was acquired. But further aspects of the learning suggest strongly that Kelli was also sensitive to the syntactic structure associated with individual verbs, and that this linguistic context is—along with the extralinguistic context—important for the discovery of verb meanings.

The Simplest Theory: Learn What You're Taught

The simplest account of Kelli's learning of *look* and *see* would be that she was explicitly taught their manual interpretations by her parents. We know that this is not so, however. Although Kelli's parents did indeed try to teach her a meaning for these verbs, it was not the meaning she learned.

The parents played a game with Kelli when she was two and three years old, in which they sang a song whose words were "Look up, Look down," and so on. They taught her to tilt her head in the appropriate spatial direction as each such command occurred in the song—in other words, to behave like the blindfolded sighted children in Experiments 1, 2, and 4 of Chapter 3. This routine was well established before Kelli was 36 months old, when our experimental work began. Under the circumstances, it is not surprising that Kelli's mother did not believe us when we told her of the outcome of the "Look up" experiments. She attributed this finding to some artifact, perhaps involving the investigator who gave the commands. Subsequently, the mother herself reran Experiment 3.1 with Kelli. The results were identical to our own: Kelli never tilted her head, but rather moved her hands, in response to *look* commands. Hence, though Kelli had learned to play a head-tilting game, her usage of *look* outside this special circumstance was always in terms of manual looking, never of visual (or head-attitude) looking. In the light of this evidence, there is no alternative but to assume that Kelli learned these words by extracting generalizations from their natural use in conversation. The question is how.

The Next Simplest Theory: Words Used in Context

Since Kelli did not acquire her uses of *look* and *see* by direct and formal inculcation, the likelihood must be that she learned these words in a naturalistic way, by observing what was going on while the words were uttered. Since Kelli's mother was the primary caregiver, our assumption was that the kind of speech and situations the mother characteristically made available must hold the answer to how Kelli learned. Therefore we set about examining videotapes in which the mother was talking to Kelli, uttering a variety of verbs including *look* and *see*. The problem was to determine how the events that accompanied the use of these words could have cued the learner to the meanings they conveyed (as documented in her speech and comprehension performances).

In an initial analysis we asked how the use of a verb is correlated with the events that were taking place and that the child could have observed (manually, of course). This analysis begins to describe how Kelli could have distinguished among various so-called motion verbs such as *give* and *get* and how she might have hit upon conjectures about their meanings. (However, this analysis will not be sufficient to describe all of Kelli's lexical acquisitions, and so will be amplified by one further analysis of the same corpus of mother-child discourse.)

Throughout the discussion (here and in Chapter 7), it is important to keep in mind that the scope of our question is herein limited to asking how the child pairs meanings (or concepts) to the verb items in her native tongue. We are not asking where the meanings or concepts come from in the first place. According to some authors (ranging from the rationalist philosophers such as Leibniz to their modern descendents such as Fodor), concepts at the appropriate level of abstractness are available to the learner from the beginning, requiring only a "triggering" by experience. Other authors (ranging from the empiricist philosophers such as Hume, Locke, and Berkeley to their many descendents in modern learning theory) suppose that the concepts are acquired by interaction with experience, through such mechanisms as association. It is not our purpose here to take a stand on these matters, though we will have some remarks to make on this topic in Chapter 9. Here we suppose only that the learner is capable—based either on "innate ideas" or on learning from the environment, we know not which—of conceiving of the notions encoded by some simple verbs. (The only theory really in opposition to this global claim is that of Whorf, 1956, who held that concepts literally derive from the language forms in some way).

We accept the general position, then, that there is a time during development when a child can implicitly conceive of the idea of 'exploring haptically' or 'perceiving haptically.' However this is accomplished, a problem remains for describing the induction of word meanings. How does the learner, so equipped, discover which of the many words she hears encodes which of the concepts she can understand? That is our only question here. Thus in the present discussion the issue of lexical concept attainment is reduced to the question—difficult enough—of how the child pairs the meanings with the correct lexical forms.

This perspective licenses a metaphoric expression we shall use throughout: The child is in possession of concepts, and her task is then to choose, among the words she hears uttered, which of them is the likely *candidate* for labelling the specific concept she has in mind.

Description of the analysis

We examined the extralinguistic and linguistic circumstances that actually accompanied Kelli's hearing of verbs. The basis for the analysis was fifteen hour-long videotaped sessions consisting largely of Kelli's interactions with her mother. These began at age 29 months, just as Kelli began to say a few simple nouns (see Table 2.1, Chapter 2). We used no tapes past the 36th month, for this is when Kelli began to use *look* and *see* spontaneously and frequently.

The logic behind the analysis is simple. If the child is learning by observing the real-world accompaniments to word use, it must be that certain words will occur when certain things are happening and can be observed by the learner. So there must be some distinguishable happenings that accompany the use of *see* which are different from the happenings for *look*, and also different from the happenings for other verbs such as *give* and *put*. The task is to find correlations between happenings and the utterance of various verbs.

Coding

The extralinguistic event

Potentially there are many ways to describe the extralinguistic situations that accompany maternal speech, ranging from physical descriptions of the situations (e.g., child's hand on target object) to very abstract ones (e.g., child in the act of exploring or seeking to explore). Our choice ultimately was based on a commonsensical view of how Kelli learned what she did. We supposed that she acquired her meanings of *look* and *see* based on a simple evidentiary source: Kelli believed *look* and *see* referred to the haptic domain because her mother used these words when Kelli was in tactual contact with target objects or close to them. Thus our assumption was that Kelli could reconstruct enough of the geometry of the ongoing scene to ascertain that some present object or person was relevant; and that if this object was located near her hands when she heard /lʌk/ this would provide a first basis for supposing that 'explore by hand' was the meaning of this verb.[1]

Accordingly, we developed the coding categories *near* (within arm's reach) and *far* (out of arm's reach) to describe Kelli's position with respect to target objects and persons, when her mother uttered verbs. (In an initial coding, an additional distinction was made between the two categories *near* and *in hand*, but this distinction turned out to do no work and so the two categories were collapsed into one.) The category *no object* was used when there was no target to observe, such as when the mother said "Let's see," musing out loud about how she (herself) was going to figure out a puzzle, or when she said "You look funny."[2]

These coding categories allow us to examine a simple view of learning verbs by ostension, that is, by observing the states of affairs that usually obtain when words are said. For the present case, we are asking if 'perceive or explore manually' is the inevitable conjecture about the meaning of *look* just because this verb, as opposed to others, occurs in maternal speech when the child is holding and manipulating some object, or at least has it within arm's reach.

The question arises how Kelli (or we) decided what the target object in the interaction might be. Sometimes things seemed easy. The mother might say "Look at Miss Barbara's boot" when Kelli was manually exploring that boot. In such cases, the linguistic circumstances (*boot* is the object of the verb *look*) and the extralinguistic circumstances (child touching a boot) conspire to yield the boot as the target object. This situation thus was assigned to the category for the use of *look* when the target object was "near."

But what if the mother said "Look at it" or even "Look" rather than "Look at the boot," when Kelli was holding or manually exploring the boot? We assumed that Kelli could usually make global inferences from the situation and the conversation. For example, while Kelli and her mother were playing with a set of stacking rings, the mother said "Look, look" and moved Kelli's hand to the rings: This was coded as "near," for the situation leads easily to the inference that the rings she had in hand and near to hand were the targets of looking, even though they are not explicitly mentioned. If the target, so defined, was more than three or four feet away from Kelli, we coded it as being "far."[3]

The linguistic event

A particular verb was assumed to have occurred whenever uttered, regardless of the syntactic construction in which it appeared and regardless of the special semantic properties that construction might imply. For example, it is possible that *look* in "You look like a kangaroo" might mean 'resemble,' i.e., this might be a case of two different verbs that happen to sound the same (for discussion of this possibility, see Chapter 7). But the assumption here is that, as learning begins, the child cannot be presumed to know that some instances of *look* encode one predicate notion while other instances encode something else.

The hypothesis under test

Our prediction was simple. If the extralinguistic circumstances caused Kelli to learn the haptic-manipulative construals, it was because the mother characteristically reserved her use of *look* and *see* to occasions when Kelli had some object (the object of the conversation as a whole or the object named in the heard sentence) in hand or near to hand, ready to be manipulated. On this hypothesis, other verbs would not occur so often in these same circumstances and so would be distinguishable from *look* and *see*.

Analysis

There were 1640 utterances in the sample. We tabulated all of those that contained perceptual verbs according to the coding scheme just described. Sixty-nine of the utterances (4 percent of all utterances) contained perceptual verbs. Fifty-two of these were *look/see* (34 instances of *look,* 18 of *see*). Other perceptual verbs (*listen, hear, watch, taste*) each occurred rarely and so were collapsed together in the tabulation. We now took a sample (roughly 33 percent of the corpus) of all other verb-containing utterances in the maternal corpus and counted instances of particular verbs. All verbs that occurred ten or more times were tabulated and coded, the rarer verbs being discarded. This left twelve common verbs: *look, see, be, come, get, give, go, have, hold, play, put,* and *say*. Their proportions in the corpus are shown in Table 6.1.

Two verbs in Table 6.1 were excluded from further analysis. The first is *say,* always used by the mother to refer to linguistic activity and in fact to induce the child to repeat, as when the mother says "Say 'thank you' to Miss Barbara" or "Say 'dog'." Both the external event and the special patterning of *say* make it easy to distinguish from all other verbs: The intonation properties of the embedded sentence or nominal are special; count nouns (e.g., *dog*) can and usually do occur in the singular without a determiner (*the*) with *say,* and so on. *Say* is the only verb in the corpus that patterns in these ways. It is the other common verbs whose distinctions from each other are harder to describe and thus will be analyzed more fully in this chapter. For related reasons, we exclude also the copula (*be*), which patterns so differently from all other items (appearance in auxiliary constructions, agreement phenomena, and so on) as to be unrealistic to include in the analyses.

Results and discussion

The major findings are presented in Table 6.2, which lists what we will call the *"near" proportion* for the various verbs, that is, the proportion of all of the mother's utterances of that verb occurring when the object was in hand or near to hand. Assuming that Kelli

Table 6.1 *Major verbs used by Kelli's mother*[a]

Verb	Proportion of total verbs
Perceptual verbs[b]	
Look	.05
See	.03
Other	.03
Total	.11
Nonperceptual verbs[b]	
Be	.28
Come	.03
Get	.04
Give	.03
Go	.03
Have	.02
Hold	.02
Play	.02
Put	.09
Say	.04
Other	.29
Total	.89

a. Major verbs were those that occurred with a frequency of 10 or greater (.01 or more) over the samples coded. "Other" is for verbs with frequency less than .01. A total of 72 verbs appeared in the sample, but only 12 occurred with sufficient frequency to count here.

b. Perceptual verbs were taken from the entire maternal corpus of 1640 utterances. This yielded 52 instances of look and see, plus 17 of other perceptual verbs combined. Nonperceptual verbs were taken from a sample of roughly 33 percent of the maternal corpus, yielding a total of 593 verbs in this analysis.

learned the meanings of *look* and *see* from this context alone, then the "near" proportion should differentiate these two verbs from all the others. We would expect to find high proportions for *look* and *see*, low proportions for the others. But as the table shows, this prediction is disconfirmed. To begin with, *look* and *see* are clearly used in different contexts by the mother, with "near" proportions of .73 and .39 respectively. A further problem is posed by the spatial contexts in which some of the other (non-sight-related) verbs were uttered. Thus *put, give,* and *hold* have higher "near" proportions than does *look* (with .97, .97, and 1.00 respectively), that for *play* is about equal (.70) to *look*, while the proportions for *have* and *go* are substantially larger than that for *see* (.53 and .52 compared to .39). All in all, there is little support for the idea that the child simply decides that the words she hears whenever an

Table 6.2 *Spatial analysis of mother's use of major verbs*

	Proportion used in contexts			
	In hand			Total number
Verb	or near	Far	No object	considered[a]
Perceptual verbs				
Look	.73	.09	.18	34
See	.39	.56	.05	18
Other perceptual	.56	.44	.00	17
Nonperceptual verbs				
Come	.05	.32	.63	19
Get	.50	.25	.25	27
Give	.97	.03	.00	21
Go	.52	.24	.24	20
Have	.53	.47	.00	11
Hold	1.00	.00	.00	10
Play	.70	.00	.30	10
Put	.97	.00	.03	61
Say	.43	.07	.50	28

a. These total to $N=276$, the number of utterances containing the common verbs (10 or more occurrences in the maternal corpus). The remaining 389 were discarded in this and following analyses, including 183 instances of *be* and 186 instances of rare verbs (fewer than 10 occurrences).

object is in her hand or nearby must refer to manual exploration or perception.

This is not to say that the spatial context here described provides no potentially useful information. It does differentiate among some of the verbs. It might for example have helped to reveal that *give* is an apposite verb to say to a person when she has an object in hand while *get* is apposite just when she doesn't. But it is clear that these spatial contexts alone will not explain how Kelli learned all that she did. For they would not alone have revealed the difference between *give* and *hold*. And they would have given her no basis for assuming that *look* and *see* are related, given the sizable difference between their "near" proportions. Nor could she have had any basis for choosing *look* rather than *put* or *hold* as the word that encodes manual exploratory activity. All she could have learned, at best, is that *get, come, go,* and *have* are wrong choices for that particular meaning.

It appears that "object nearby" (as coded by the "near" proportion) is an insufficient basis for the full set of inductions about verb meaning that we know Kelli made. One might argue that we chose the wrong contextual criterion—that a geometrical layout of the scene, with objects located relative to the child listener, was not the way in which Kelli encoded the context (or it was not particularly salient). If so, then our results have no bearing on the contextual learning hypothesis, for the only contextual encoding that can be relevant to language learning is the learner's own.

This argument is surely too drastic, however. Kelli, like all young language learners, was certainly able to perceive and note where objects were in relation to her body. Such locational distinctions are in fact encoded in a large subset of the common verbs of all languages: the so-called motion verbs, which describe the positions, paths, and goals of entities that move through space in various ways. As an example, consider *give* and *get*. A spatial-locational analysis of these verbs asserts that in the sentence

(1) John gives a book to Mary,

an entity (book) starts out near a person (John) and moves so as to end up far from that person (i.e., near Mary). In the sentence

(2) Mary gets a book from John,

an entity (book) starts out far from a person (Mary) and moves so as to end up near that person (far from John). What is interesting is that this description of the spatial displacement pattern does fit the contexts in which Kelli heard *give* and *get* and thus may be relevant to how she learned their meanings. As Table 6.2 shows, *give* but not *get* was almost invariably used when the child had the relevant object in hand or near to hand when the action began.

We believe, then, that the coding categories chosen were relevant. But another objection may be raised to them: Perhaps they encode the motional aspects of the observed scenes in a way that is less "abstract" than the encodings used by children, Kelli in particular. Good candidates for more abstract coding categories are those that figure in the semantic-relation sentence descriptions favored by many psychologists (or the thematic-role descriptions of predicate-argument structures favored by many linguists). Such descriptions organize the world in terms of a scenario in which some predicate idea (*give*) is related to a set of arguments of that predicate: the giver, or *agent*, the givee, or *recipient*, and that which is given, or *patient*. In this alternative terminology the description of *give* in sentence (1) involves the movement of a *patient* (that which is given) from the *source* at which giving starts (John) to a *goal* at which giving is accomplished (Mary). For *get* in sentence (2), there is motion of a *patient* (that which is gotten) to a *goal* (Mary) from a *source* (John).

We have no strong opinion concerning whether the coding categories for the various verb arguments should have been labelled "source" rather than "near," and the like, though it is surely harder to relate the more abstract categories to the real observables in the child's experiential world. If the reader prefers the abstract labels, he should feel free to substitute them for the "near" and "far" categories. The point is that this will make no difference at all in describing the correlations betwen verb use and situations (so encoded). This is because *near* and *source* cover exactly the same situations, *far* and *goal* cover exactly the same situations, and *target object* and *patient* cover exactly the same situations. The labels change, but the correlations do not. Therefore the label choices are no more than a matter of taste with respect to how they will map onto the descriptions of the events accompanying Kelli's hearing of the various verbs.

In sum, the coding categories used in the present analysis are equivalent to the standard semantic-relational descriptions of sentential logic in the sense that they make the same distinctions in describing the same external situations. We prefer our own terms only because they avoid mental characterizations of the event presented to the child learner (we do not wish to take a stand as to whether these are somehow "observable"), emphasizing instead the physical characteristics of the situation (which surely are observable).

It has just been argued that the spatial coding choices were relevant, for they reflect the fact that children can observe the relative locations of entities in space, and in a way that will map quite simply onto the predicate-argument structure of sentences the child ultimately learns to say and understand. These spatial contexts differentiate the meanings of some simple motion verbs in the mother's speech. This is of some interest because the case of *give* and *get*—common in the mother's speech and evidently easily acquired by Kelli—seems at first inspection to be a difficult one. The difficulty is that these two verbs describe all and only the same scenes in the observable world. Every situation of giving is a situation of getting as well: Whenever John gives Mary a book, it is also true that Mary gets a book from John.[4]

The meanings of *give* and *get* can be pried apart only if the observer is capable of taking a particular perspective on the scene— who has the object when action begins and who has it when action is completed. Our coding scheme incorporated this perspective by making the assumption that Kelli could determine the target object (the object moved) and its movement when verbs occurred in sentences addressed to her (from near to far from her in the case of *give* and from far to near to her in the case of *get*).

Thus the codings chosen for describing the event seem natural enough and may partly account for what was learned.[5]

A Syntactically Controlled Analysis

Though the spatial-locational analysis had some success in accounting for the acquisition of motion verbs, clearly it did not answer to how Kelli acquired the meanings of *look* and *see*. We shall now try to show that use of the spatial-locational categories of experience taken together with a more sophisticated scheme for analyzing heard sentences can account for how Kelli individuated the full set of frequent verbs she heard.

In the prior analysis, it was granted only that the child could hear and isolate some sound signal, such as /lʌk/, and that she would then attempt to correlate the occurrence of this signal with the location and movement of persons and objects. Thus the form/meaning pairing that in Chapter 1 we asserted was the necessary condition for learning was first assumed to be extracted from a *word/event* input pair. In the analysis now to be presented, it is supposed that the child also knows where these sound signals occur in sentences. Thus the form/meaning pairing is now assumed to be extracted from a *sentence/event* input pair. Specifically, we now conjecture that the child, while inspecting the scene before her, is considering the verb, say /lʌk/, *as it appears in a syntactic structure.*

Is there any reason to believe that the very young child we are investigating, learning her first simple verbs and sentences, would have access to syntactic analyses? The evidence from language-acquisition research amply demonstrates that children do have linguistic information that was not exploited in our previous analysis: Learners can perform global syntactic parsings of sentences early in life. They can organize the string of words into sequenced, hierarchically arranged phrasal categories, based on an analysis of such perceptual properties of the wave form as accent, tone, and vocalic length (for the evidence that children at the earliest stages of language acquisition perform such analyses, see Chapter 7; for a fuller statement, see Gleitman and Wanner, 1982, 1984). It is now assumed that the learner represents the utterances heard in terms of the parse trees that can be derived from such analyses.[6]

Examples of these parse trees are shown in Figure 6.1, which provides the standard phrasal description of sentences containing *give* and *get*. This global description of the sentence analyzes it into phrase categories such as noun-phrase (NP), verb-phrase (VP),

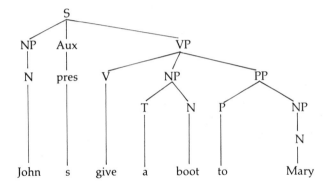

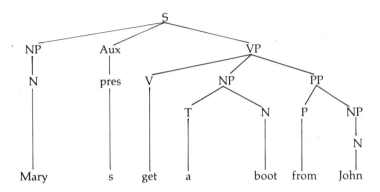

Figure 6.1 *Phrase–structural descriptions of sentences with* give *and* get. *(For technical reasons of no great interest in the present context, the auxiliary material—the present-tense marker—is represented as preceding the verb in these diagrams.)*

prepositional phrase (PP), and the like. Each of these categories is further analyzed in terms of such lexical categories as noun (N), verb (V), preposition (P), and so forth. We are now supposing that this is the representational format in terms of which the child analyzes the utterances she hears. And it is against this format that she considers the contexts of use (analyzed, as before, by the spatial-locational scheme).

This new stance represents a radical upgrading of the information basis hypothetically granted to learners. To see why, consider Figure 6.2, which represents the phrasal analysis of two sentences that actually occurred in the maternal corpus: *Let's see Miss Bar-*

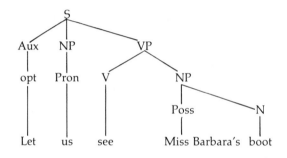

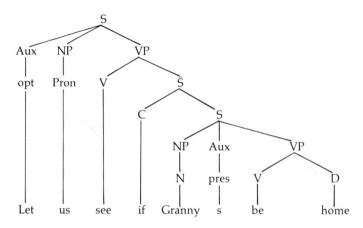

Figure 6.2 *Panel 1 shows a sentence from the maternal corpus in which* see *occurs with a simple NP object. Panel 2 shows a sentence from the maternal corpus in which* see *occurs with a following NP, but that NP is embedded in a complement clause.*

bara's boot and *Let's see if Granny is home.* Note that the second sentence is analyzed in Figure 6.2 as containing an embedded sentence (*if Granny is home*) while the first sentence is not. An NP that follows the verb *see* (*Granny* and *Miss Barbara's boot*) thus may be organized within the sentence in quite different ways: The NP *Granny* is embedded in an internal sentence, while the NP *Miss Barbara's boot* is not. As we will show, this distinction will be relevant to why the child will believe the boot must be near if *see* is to mean what it does, but Granny need not be near even though *see* means what it does.

Summarizing, the claim now made is that the learner, at some language-developmental stage earlier than investigated here, has extracted the major lexical and phrasal categories of the language being learned, and can construct global surface parses of sentences in which these categories are the labels. These parses, along with the analysis of the spatial position of objects in the extralinguistic scene, are assumed to enter into the task of learning the meanings of verbs.

The hypothesis under test

Our prediction was that the verbs as used by Kelli's mother would be distinctive in their syntactic environments, providing a format within which their meanings could be individuated. Further, we predicted as in the prior analysis that the spatial-locational coding of the situation of use (*near, far, no object*) would provide trustworthy information about the meanings, but now only as constrained by the syntactic structure of the mother's sentences.

Coding

Each utterance containing one of the verbs listed in Table 6.2 was coded according to its *subcategorization frame*. The subcategorization frame of a verb is a description of the phrasal categories (such as NP or PP) that appear following a verb and that represent the arguments of the predicate. For example, in the sentence *John saw Mary*, an NP (*Mary*) follows the verb. The subcategorization frames do not indicate the structure preceding the verb, for this is always the same regardless of the verb—an NP representing the subject of the sentence. In contrast, verbs differ in the phrasal material that follows them. For example, we say that *banish* occurs in the frame "——— NP" because this verb requires an NP following it (one can say "John banished the rabbit" but not *"John banished," *"John banished up," or *"John banished to the table"). In contrast, we say that *vanish* occurs in the frame "——— Ø" because one can say "The rabbit vanished" but not e.g., *"John vanished the rabbit."[7]

It is not always easy to determine the subcategorization frame, given an utterance. For example, in a sentence like *John relied on Mary*, it is necessary to say that *on Mary* is part of the required structural material associated with this verb, in part because without it (**John relied*) the sentence is not grammatical. But in *John sang in Mexico* there are reasons to suppose that *in Mexico* is no part of the argument structure but is only an optional PP of the kind that can occur with any verb (the sentence is still grammatical if this PP is removed; the PP can appear preceding the subject NP, and so on). But there are some cases that are not so easy. In the sentence *John*

Table 6.3 *Subcategorization frames for the common verbs*

	Group I		Group II				Group III			
	Look[a]	See[a]	Give[a]	Put[a]	Hold[a]	Play	Get[a]	Have	Go[a]	Come[a]
Look/see only										
Deictic										
V!	8									
V?		1								
V!, S	10									
V?, S		3								
V rel$_{how}$	2									
Other										
V like NP	5									
V S		5					1[b]			
come V NP		3								
Exclude *look/see*										
V NP PP			5	31	1		2			
V NP D				28	6		2			
V D NP				1						
V NP NP			16				2			
V rel$_{where}$				1						
Overlap with *look/see*										
V PP	3					7[c]			2	2
V D	2						5		10	13
V Ø	2	3							8	4
V NP		3			3	3	13	14		
V AP	2						3			
Totals	34	18	21	61	10	10	27	15	20	19

a. Verbs that occur with locative prepositions and adverbs.

b. A causative use of *have:* "Will we have Barbara come baby sit?"

c. *Play* with the nonlocative (reciprocal) preposition *with:* "You're not gonna play with the triangle, so forget it!"

played with blocks there is some question whether *with blocks* should be analyzed as part of the predicate material or is an optional adjoined phrase. Since these questions are real, two independent judges coded all of the utterances. Their judgments were in accord for over .95 of the utterances.[8]

Analysis and findings

This analysis was performed on the same corpus of 1640 utterances spoken by the mother in Kelli's presence before the age of 36 months, that is, before the meanings of *look* and *see* were established as shown by her speech and comprehension performances.

Only the frequent verbs, as listed in Table 6.2, were considered in the analysis.

Subcategorization frames for the frequent verbs

In Table 6.3 is shown the number of times each verb occurred in a particular subcategorization frame. Table 6.3 thus indicates the verb occurrences in the maternal corpus according to these syntactic subcategorizations. In addition, the individual verbs appear in the table as organized by the prior analysis (Table 6.2): *look* and *see* constitute Group I; Group II consists of all other frequent verbs that appeared over two-thirds of the time in the "near" condition; those in Group III fell more often into the "far" and "no object" categories.

Inspection of Table 6.3 reveals that the frequent verbs have highly distinctive syntactic privileges of occurrence, in terms of the subcategorization frames they allow. As one example, the mother does produce such utterances as "Put the baby doll on the shelf" but not "Look the baby doll on the shelf." Such distinctions of syntactic format for various verbs are well known to be characteristic of adult-to-adult language use. But what is important here is that these distinctive syntactic patterns show up clearly even in our relatively small sample of maternal speech. Thus if a learner is disposed to do so, she can inspect these syntactic patterns to gain information about the individual verbs. Consider the major patterns of syntactic format that are tabulated in Table 6.3. The first rows of the table show syntactic environments in which only *look* and *see* occur. A subset of these environments is restricted to *see*:

(1) Only *see* appears in deictic interjective queries ("See?" and "See?, That's a circle").

(2) With a single exception, only *see* appears with sentential complements ("Let's see if Granny's home").[9]

Another set of environments is restricted to *look*:

(3) Only *look* appears in deictic interjective commands ("Look!" and "Look, That's a boot").

(4) Only *look* appears deictically with a free *how* relative ("Look how I do it").

(5) Only *look* appears in constructions with *like* ("You look like a kangaroo in those overalls").

Thus *look* and *see* are in some ways distinct from all other verbs and distinct from each other.

A second group of the frequent verbs appears in syntactic environments which are disallowed for *look* and *see* (as well as *come, go, play,* and *have*):

(6) *Look* and *see* allow a maximum of two associated NPs, Ds, and PPs, while other verbs may (*get, hold*) or must (*give, put*) take three of these: English allows *Mary gives John the book, Mary holds the book out,* and *Mary puts the book on the table. Look* and *see* do not occur in such environments (**Mary sees the book to John*), nor do such verbs as *come* (**Mary comes the horse to John*).

One further pattern is notable in Table 6.3:

(7) Most of the verbs occurred in the corpus with a range of locative prepositions and adverbs, but *have* and *play* did not. Specifically, *have* occurs with an NP object, never taking a locative of any kind (*She has one of the rings* but not **She has down one of the rings*). *Play* occurs characteristically (seven out of ten times) with the nonlocative (reciprocal) preposition *with,* as in *Don't play with that spoon,* and disallows locative prepositions used adverbially (**Let's play Monopoly up*) except in idiomatic constructions that never appeared in the data base (*all played out, She played up her importance,* and so on).[10]

As we have stated, with a few exceptions the restrictive patterns just discussed are characteristic of ordinary speech, not only of the present sample corpus. We shall show in Chapter 7 that these distinctive syntactic encodings for the various common verbs are interestingly, though complexly, correlated with their semantic properties.

Look/see in the near/far environments as a function of their syntactic frames

Recall that a particular problem of Analysis 1 was the very poor predictive power of the spatial coding categories for *see* (.39 "near" proportion) and the relatively poor predictive power for *look* (.73 "near" proportion) compared with *give* (97 percent "near" proportion). Table 6.4 shows the spatial analysis for these two verbs again, but this time within syntactic subcategorization frames. Though the number of entries in each cell in the table now becomes quite small, and thus may not be reliable, more reasonable patterns of "near" proportions do seem to emerge.

Consider first the entries under Row 1 of the table. These show the maternal uses of *look* and *see* in their canonical subcategorization frames ("look at NP," "look D," "see NP") and the deictic interjective uses that are the most frequent in the maternal corpus (e.g., "Look!" and "See? That's a frog"). When these syntactic

Table 6.4 *The spatial analysis of* look *and* see

	Near	Far	No object	"Near" proportion
Canonical sentence frames and deictic uses				
Look at NP	3	0	0	
Look D	2	0	0	1.00
Look!	8	0	0	
Look! this is NP	10	0	0	
See NP	1	2	0	
See?	1	0	0	.72
See?, This is NP	3	0	0	
With motion auxiliaries				
Come see NP	0	3	0	.00
Other environments				
Look AP	0	1	1	
Look like NP	0	0	5	.18
Look how$_{rel}$	0	2	0	
Look Ø	2	0	0	
See S	2	3	0	.25
See Ø	0	2	1	
Total (all environments)				
Look	25	3	6	.73
See	7	10	1	.39

types only are considered, the "near" proportion for *look* rises to 1.00 (from .73 in Table 6.2), and that for *see* rises to .72 (from .39).

The entries under Row 2 show the maternal uses of *see* with *come* and *go* as auxiliary verbs (e.g., "Let's go see Granny"). As it happens, *look* does not occur in the sample corpus in this construction, though there is no syntactic prohibition against it. For such constructions the "near" proportion of *see* is zero.

The entries under Row 3 show a variety of further formats in which these two verbs occurred in the corpus. These are (1) intransitive uses ("I see," "Let's look"), (2) uses of *look* with adjectival and adverbial phrases ("You look funny," "You look like a hunchback"), (3) uses of *see* with sentential complements ("Let's see if Granny is coming"), and (4) uses of *look* with free *how* relatives ("Let's see how you do it"). For these categories taken as a group, the "near" proportion is .18 and .25 for *look* and *see* respectively.

Thus, though we reemphasize that the number of cases per cell

Table 6.5 *How Kelli's mother used* look *and* see

In haptic context
    a. Where "feel" seems directly intended:
      "Let's look at this." (K is fingering a form board)
    b. As attention getter, but "feel" is an easy interpretation:
      "Look, Miss Barbara's boot." (guiding K's hands over boot)
      "Look, here's how you wind the clock."

Out of haptic context
    "See camera." (repetition of K's request to "see camera")
    "Come see the kitty." (cat is at a distance)
    "Gonna go see Granny and Poppy?" (meaning, go to their house)

Amodal
    a. Find out, by other than visual or haptic means:
      "Let's see if Granny's home, ok?" (dialing telephone)
      "Let's see: what kind of cheese do you want?"
      "See if you can put the slipper on."
    b. Where mother probably had in mind a construal that requires vision, but where some nonvisual, or amodal, construal seems possible:
      "She looks beautiful." (said of a doll K is holding)
      "You look like a kangaroo." (K is wearing overalls with a pouch)
      "You look funny."
      "You look like a hunchback."

in this new breakdown is small, it does appear that the failure of the spatial analysis for *look* and *see* is restricted to certain syntactic environments. And the syntactic analysis is hardly arbitrary. Inspected more closely, it is coherent with what the mother evidently meant by the verbs, as it apparent both from their syntactic forms and from observation of the situations in which they were used (for samples, see Table 6.5). The interjective uses of the visual verbs ("Look!" and "See?") were intended, roughly, as attention getters, requesting the child to explore or attend to objects. The canonical uses with NP objects again usually described, queried, or commanded the exploration or apprehension of nearby objects, and the canonical uses of *look* with a locative adverb ("Look around," "Look down," "Look over there") requested the child to attend to certain locations. It is in these uses that target objects were generally near the child listener. In contrast, the maternal utterances with *come* and *go* auxiliaries ("Come look at this") were uttered while the child was far from an object for reasons that are transparent. The uses with sentential objects were intended to encode comments, requests, or commands to observe an event, rather than a concrete object. Intransitives were characteristically used by the mother when musing aloud about a problem or choice ("Hmm . . . Let's see"). The use of "look like" and "look AP" were intended in the sense of 'resemble.'

Removing these offending interpretations on the basis of their distinctive linguistic encoding yields stable uses of both *look* and *see* in extralinguistic circumstances (object in hand or nearby) that would be supportive of the conjectures Kelli made about their meanings: that they pertain to the haptic exploration and perception of objects. Thus if it is believed that Kelli performed the syntactic pre-analysis of Table 6.4, concentrating on the extralinguistic circumstances for selected syntactic environments—the deictic uses and the canonical subcategorization frames for these verbs—she was in a position to make the induction that *look* and *see* had something to do with the "nearby-ness" of target objects and therefore are both at least candidates for the construal 'explore manually.'

Discussion

We have attempted to describe the conditions under which Kelli acquired her meanings for *look* and *see*. The first analysis asked whether these words occur in a patterned way as a function of scenes in the world. This analysis failed for *look* and *see*, and in our opinion it was foredoomed. It might have been realistic to hope, given only the weakest constraints on the human representational and perceptual system, that construals like those for action verbs such as *tickle, bite,* and *smack* might leap out at the learner as the only salient choices after a modest number of exposures to their real-world uses, though the failure of the spatial-locational analysis to distinguish among *put, hold,* and *give* (all of which had about the same "near" proportion) shows that even for simple verbs of physical motion no very superficial—or inevitable—analysis of the event will answer to the detailed and highly articulated verb meanings that a young child acquires. Moreover, as is clear at least in retrospect, no inevitable inductions about the meanings of verbs like *look* and *see* (or *know, think, pretend, lie, want, hope, need,* etc.) which involve mental states, goals, and apprehensions, could reasonably fall out of simple correlations between real-world events and the utterance of words.

Therefore we attempted in a second analysis to limit the work that the environmental circumstances would have to do, placing part of the burden of learning elsewhere. We were able to demonstrate that a child equipped with the capacity and inclination to examine the syntactic format of each sentence was in a position to distinguish among the common verbs (Table 6.3). Moreover, the learner could then extract certain linguistic environments within which the spatial analysis of events would include *look* and *see* among those likely to occur when a target object is nearby (Table 6.4). This was important if the child was to entertain the idea that these verbs pertained to haptic exploration, which can take place only on objects within arm's reach.

But despite these apparent descriptive successes, our analyses do not speak directly to two central problems in accounting for lexical concept attainment. We reintroduce these problems here to show the limits on what has so far been explained and to set the stage for further discussion in Chapters 7 and 9.

"Salient" interpretations of scenes and events

All of our analyses have presupposed (rather than explained) that Kelli was likely to entertain the hypothesis that there would be verbs in the maternal corpus appropriate for encoding the notions 'haptic exploration' (*look*) and 'haptic perception' (*see*). In contrast, we assumed that Kelli would not be seeking a construal for certain unlikely meanings, such as 'head tilt' ('orient the head in various spatial directions relative to the trunk'). Indeed, as we have described, the parents tried to teach this idea in the context of a song and the child rejected the chance to learn it; at least she did not transfer this usage outside the song context. Perhaps it can be argued that 'head tilt' had no utility for Kelli in her everyday life and that this is why she failed to learn it. But it is not always so easy to understand the properties of the lexical concepts she did and did not attain.

As a more realistic example, then, let us ask why Kelli (and the sighted control subjects) learned modality-tied rather than amodal interpretations for *look* and *see*. Their experiences must support either of these interpretations; i.e., every experience of 'perceive visually' (or, in Kelli's case, 'perceive manually') is also a case of 'perceive.' Surely 'perceive' is a concept that has utility, and it is supported in experience as well as is 'perceive manually.' Why do the child learners reject the "higher-level" categorizations in favor of the "lower-level" ones? For that matter, why don't they choose yet lower-level construals of these same scenes? Why didn't Kelli learn that *look* means 'move the hand to' (i.e., that it means the same as *touch*) since every experience, for her, of exploring the world haptically is also an experience of moving the hand to an object?

In our view, the problem in understanding acquisition of the verb meanings is not so much that no basis for the correct inductions is available from the environments of use. As we have shown, a syntactically constrained set of observations of the external events is consistent with what was learned. The more difficult problem is that there is a basis for very many kinds of induction; in each case all but one of them wrong. In short, a hidden presupposition of all our analyses is that the child would limit her search for word meaning to realistic and salient parsings of the world of objects and events. We will later (Chapter 9) take up the topic of how these limits might be imposed by the child learner. In the present context, it is important to notice that this crucial problem has been finessed rather than engaged in the analyses presented.

Can syntactic analysis support semantic analysis?

Analysis 2 showed that the frequent verbs Kelli heard can be distinguished from each other by attention to the syntactic formats in which they occur. But a question this analysis leaves aside is really the one of major interest: What good are these distinguishing *syntactic* properties for a child who is trying to discover the *meanings* of words? Can the available extralinguistic and linguistic contexts support Kelli's conjecture that *look* and *see* pertain to haptic exploration and perception, differ from each other in that one describes an activity and the other describes a mental state, and so on? Grossly, it seems that the prospects are good. For example, it is obvious to the point of banality that *go look* should take off the "nearby-ness" requirement for the use of *look*, for a learner subtle enough to notice it. Moreover, the fact that *see* takes sentential complements is consistent with the fact that it can label the perception of events as well as the perception of concrete objects. In general, there seems to be some initial support for the idea that the internal syntactic distinctions among verbs hold promise for discoveries about the meanings of the predicates they encode.

7 / Syntactic and Ostensive Supports for Verb Learning

The purpose to which we now turn is to explain Kelli's—and all children's—acquisition of a verb lexicon. The thrust of the analyses of Chapter 6 was that the external events that accompany speech comprise only one of several contributory sources of information for the discovery of verb meanings. Specifically, clues in the surface forms of utterances spoken to Kelli were sufficient to distinguish each of the frequent verbs from all the others: These were the differing syntactic subcategorization frames for each verb. The question raised now is whether these distinctive properties of form can help the learner select the meaning properties of verbs. We shall argue from an inspection of the correlations between verb forms and their meanings that syntactic structure is at least in principle an informative source of evidence for the young learner.

It should be kept in mind that, just as before, we are not seeking to explain where such concepts as 'move an object from a source to a goal' or 'explore haptically' come from. Maybe some coherence can be given to the idea that they come as original equipment with the neonate rather than being learned at all. Or maybe some coherent theory can be developed that shows how they are acquired by familiar mechanisms of learning. We assume only that these concepts are acquired *somehow,* accounting for Kelli's speech and comprehension performances with the various verbs. Again our question is how Kelli decided which of the many verbs she heard are paired with each of these presupposed concepts. As remarked earlier, this problem is hard enough. And we will now try to show that this problem, like all hard ones, requires an intricate answer.

Speaking particularly, we now pursue the idea that the child's verb learning is facilitated by her attention to the syntactic organization of the sentences she hears. One suggestive though indirect particle of evidence for such a conjecture is worth noting at the outset. As Lenneberg (1967) showed, there is usually a period at the very beginning of language development when the acquisition of vocabulary is slow and effortful. This is roughly the period ending at the second birthday. Three developments begin at about this time. The child's vocabulary, heretofore restricted primarily to concrete nouns such as *table* (see Chapter 2), expands to include more verbs and adjectives; the rate of word learning increases dramatically, to about five to seven words a day; at the same time, rudimentary syntax (two-word utterances) appears in the child's speech repertoire. Our suggestion is that these advances are intimately connected: Verb learning, while partly a function of the ostensive evidence provided, feeds upon the conceptual representation of predicate-argument logic in the syntactic format of the sentence. Thus when the child gives evidence of controlling some of this logic, word learning is greatly facilitated.[1]

The following discussion proceeds in four steps. First we consider what the learner brings into the verb-learning task by reviewing evidence about the earliest stages of language learning. Second we describe the semantic inferences that a learner could make—given that she has a limited number of plausible candidate meanings in mind—by inspecting the subcategorization frames for common verbs in the mother's speech. In particular, we ask which inferences would in principle have been available to Kelli from inspection of the maternal corpus as analyzed in Chapter 6. As may be obvious in advance, such a discussion is dependent upon a general characterization of the way that verbs are represented in the mental lexicon (of adults as well as child learners). Third, therefore, we propose a description of the verb lexicon; this proposal is orthodox in part but has some novel properties. Finally, a general discussion tries to bring together these strands so as to propose strategies for verb learning.

What the Learner Brings
to the Verb-Learning Task

Where is the learner to begin the quest for the relations between sound and meaning? We first review evidence concerning the knowledge that young learners bring into the task of learning verb meanings. (1) They seem to have at least rudimentary conceptual knowledge of the logical forms of sentences (predicate-argument structures) and are disposed to believe that nominals encode the arguments and verbs encode the predicates in such structures. (2) They can construct surface parses (phrase structural analyses) of the sentences they hear, which may serve as the representational formats on which detailed verb inductions are performed. The verb-learning scenario we shall try to defend depends on both these kinds of supposition about the child's initial state.

Initial conceptual representations

Conceptions underlying major form-class distinctions

Many investigators (Slobin, 1981; Gentner, 1982; Braine and Hardy, 1982; Pinker, 1982, 1984; and many other sources) suggest that we must begin by granting two rather strong (and not so self-evident) conjectures to the learner. The first is that verbs encode actions and states, and the second is that nouns encode persons, places, and things. This claim is certainly not that these fourth-grade definitions of the syntactic classes describe mature language knowledge. It is rather that these are initial conjectures by means of which the child bootstraps his way toward the major lexical classes (formal distributional analysis later can add such nonactions as *seem* to the set of verbs and such nonthings as *justice* to the set of nouns; see Maratsos, 1982).[2]

A first indication of this distinction appears in the properties of the child's first rudimentary sentences (produced at about two years of age; see Figures 2.2 and 2.3). These usually consist only of two words: a noun and a verb. As has been shown repeatedly, this noun and verb differ in their serial ordering in the young child's utterances in languages like English (Bloom, 1970; Brown, 1973; Slobin, 1973; Maratsos, 1982), or—in other languages—by the inflectional markers they select (e.g., Hebrew: see Levy, 1983b), or both (e.g., Serbo-Croatian: see Slobin, 1982).

Evidence that this noun/verb distinction comes in part from the child's preexisting biases about the nature of a language, rather than from transparent inductions over the input corpus, has been presented by Feldman, Goldin-Meadow, and Gleitman (1978; Goldin-Meadow, 1982), who studied deaf children of hearing parents who were not exposed to sign language and could not learn a spoken language owing to their deafness. As apparently often occurs with children in these circumstances, they developed manual communication systems (called "home sign" by the deaf community). Even in these informal and untutored systems, the investigators were able to show that nouns and verbs were distinguished both in their form (the kind of iconic gesture used) and in their syntactic organization (their position in gestured sentences).

We cannot say exactly how learners exposed to ordinary language data make the initial decision about which morphological items are to be the nouns (and thus encode the persons and objects) and which are to be the verbs (and thus encode the actions and states), but see Pinker, 1984, for discussion. Perhaps special properties of ostension and of the forms of maternal utterances (e.g., *That's* a man; he's *jumping*) can be shown to bear on this problem (Shipley, Kuhn, and Madden, 1983). But however it is accomplished, this partitioning of the lexical stock has already been made at the moment in development we are concerned with: when the child begins to determine the meanings of the various verbs.

The predicate-argument analysis of sentences

Gleitman and Wanner have reviewed evidence showing that the young learner is predisposed to consider the sentence of English in terms of a predicate-argument logic in which the verb serves as the predicate itself and the various nominals surrounding it serve as its arguments. Evidence comes from an examination of young children's speech. At early stages of language learning, with only rare exceptions, each of the formatives (separate lexical items) in the child's speech encodes (a) a predicate, (b) an argument of that predicate, or (c) a logical word such as *not*. Words that serve other functions, such as auxiliary verbs, relativizers, determiners, and adjectives, are largely missing from speech during a lengthy period during development.

Most revealing, according to Gleitman and Wanner, it is occasionally true of language as used by mature individuals that some of these relational and logical items are conflated within a single formative. For instance, *not* is conflated within the subject NP for certain indefinite pronominals of standard English: We say "Nobody likes me," not "Anybody (or nobody) does *not* like me." But young children, including Kelli (see Chapter 5), resist such conflations, saying "Anybody can't see me now" or "Nobody don't like me" often despite strenuous attempts of their parents to correct them (McNeill, 1966; for further documentation, see Newport, 1982). Summarizing, the young learner seems to be predisposed to organize the sentence structure by uttering words that figure directly in the predicate-argument logic—the words that would be the heads of the semantically functioning phrases in adult well-formed sentences—omitting all else.

In addition, learners seem to know how many arguments a particular verb intent requires, without instruction (though they could not know their placement within syntactic structures, for this varies for the predicates of a single language and varies extensively across languages). One source of evidence is again the deaf isolates. Feldman et al. were able to show by a syntactic analysis of these children's gestured sentences that they conceived a single argument for a verb such as *sleep* (the experiencer of the action) and so used only a single nominal with this verb; but they conceived two arguments for *hit* (the agent and patient), providing it with two nominal phrases, and three arguments for *give* (agent, patient, recipient), providing it with three nominal phrases in their signed sentences. We shall assume that children exposed to ordinary language data have the same presuppositions: that the logic of a predicate such as *give* involves the one who gives, the one who is given, and the thing that is given, while *sleep* involves only its experiencer. In Chapter 6 it was shown that this analysis—at least for the common verbs of motion—can be constructed in terms of the positions and motions of objects relative to the learner's body (and can be mapped onto the linguistic formatives by attention to syntactic structure).

Which predicates are lexicalized? Finally, the deaf subjects of Feldman et al. also document a point so self-evident that usually we do not notice that it *requires* documentation. Without formal linguistic exposure, children suppose that certain ideas are worth lexicalizing (e.g., 'sleep,' 'hit', 'give') while many others are not (e.g., the absurd and complex idea of 'either singing or leaking out of containers', cf. Osherson, 1978). The topic of "natural" versus "absurd" lexical choices will concern us in Chapter 9. Here it suffices to point out that the learner must bring some such biases into the learning situation. As we have remarked before, only such presuppositions can ultimately account for why 'head tilting' seems never to be considered as the construal for *look*—either for sighted children, who in principle could so encode each experience they have with this word, or for Kelli, who was deliberately tutored in this construal.

In particular, the analyses of Chapter 6 suggest some of the categories that are recruited in language learning. Kelli seems to have made use of the spatial locations and motions of objects in her environment as the experiental basis for reconstructing predicate-argument structures. If so, the tendency to observe the world according to the positions and motions of objects in space is part of the equipment the child (blind or sighted) brings into the learning situation. We pointed to experimental demonstrations of Kelli's spatial knowledge beginning earlier than any language knowledge

(Landau et al., 1981, 1984) as support for the idea that even a blind child can encode her environment spatially.

Syntactic representations

We have attempted to show that the verbs cannot be individuated *solely* by inspecting the real-world situation that accompanies their use, even if it is granted that this situation is naturally conceived in ways relevant to the construction of predicate-argument logic. We proposed that acquisition of the meanings of verbs requires also that the learner make reference to a linguistic analysis of heard sentences, their parse structures. But if this is so, it must be that the child has access to this parse for the sake of learning, rather than arriving at this parse as the outcome of learning. A crucial question, then, is whether the learner has a basis for constructing the surface parse before the verbs are individuated and hence before the whole ball game is over. We presupposed this in Chapter 6, but we now present evidence that exists in its support.

Gleitman and Wanner reviewed evidence that phrase-structure analyses of heard sentences can be constructed by young learners on the basis of sentence prosody. Their initial information is derived in large from a bottom-up, perceptually automatic analysis of the speech wave in terms of the physical analysis underlying such segmental categories as *stressed syllable* and *lengthened syllable* and such suprasegmental categories as *rhythmicity* and *tone*. Syntactic as well as lexical factors influence the way these properties are manifested in the sound patterns of spoken sentences. For example, pauses and durational patterns (syllable length) in the wave form are fine-grained enough to pick out syntactic constituents and even to distinguish syntactic boundaries of varying strengths (Klatt, 1975, 1976; Liberman and Streeter, 1976; Nakatani and Dukes, 1977; Nakatani and Schaffer, 1978; Streeter, 1978; Cooper and Paccia-Cooper, 1980). These distinguishing physical properties can be expected to be even more obvious in maternal speech to young children, which is slower in overall rate and more exaggerated in prosodic contours (Fernald and Simon, 1984).

A significant body of evidence supports the idea that learners exploit these physical clues. Fernald (1982, 1984) has shown that infants prefer to listen to the exaggerated contours of Motherese (the special style characteristic of adult-to-child speech) rather than to adult-to-adult talk. Obviously this has nothing to do with the meaning of the Motherese discourse, for infants understand not a word of it. Spring and Dale (1977) have shown discrimination of linguistic stress in early infancy. Babbling in the prespeech period already shows language-specific choices among these categories (DeBoysson-Bardies, Sagart, and Durand, 1984). Early free speech (Gleitman and Wanner, 1982) and imitative speech (Blasdell and Jensen, 1970) reproduce the same salient properties of the wave form. Read and Schreiber (1982) among others have shown that older children can extract and report syntactic constituents (e.g., subject of the sentence) based on these prosodic cues. Finally, these generalizations about prosodic influences on language learning hold true across languages where the grammatical and semantic functions assigned by particular prosodic properties differ (Slobin, 1982; Pye, 1983; Mithun, forthcoming; and see Gleitman and Wanner for this analysis, based on the cross-linguistic evidence presented by the authors just cited).

Summary

Accepting the evidence just summarized, we suppose that children approach the problem of individuating the verb meanings armed with a vocabulary of simple concrete nouns, and at least rudimentary conceptual understanding of predicate-argument logic and its mapping onto the spatial properties of scenes. Learners also have biases about at least some simple predicates and substantives that are natural to lexicalize. Moreover, they can construct a surface parse of utterances heard and can place the verb within this parse on the prosodic evidence.

All this prior apparatus granted, we now return to the problem of how a child might learn which verbs encode which meanings. For after all, we have only reviewed evidence that on hearing "The ball rolls off the table" the child can parse it roughly as

$$_S(_{NP} \text{ (the ball)}_{VP}(_V(\text{rolls})_{PP}(\text{off}_{NP}(\text{the table}))))$$

How does she decide on the meaning of the verb?

Interacting Syntactic and Ostensive Cues to Verb Meaning

Inspection of linguistic structures could contribute to the discovery of verb meaning if it is really true that these structures are reflections of the meanings they encode. But stated in so general a way, this position is not even controversial. Consider, for example, sentences containing the word *put*; these always require three noun-phrases as in *John put the book on the table*. This is no arbitrary syntactic fact about *put* but rather is a consequence of the fact that this predicate is used to describe the activity of some agent (in this case, John) who moves some object (the book) to some location (the table). It is a fact about the way language encodes events that predicts this structure if a verb is to mean what *put* means. In contrast, the semantics of *laugh* assure that sentences like *John laughed the soup on the table* are close to incomprehensible (and that *John laughed the proposal off the table* is metaphorical). Interestingly enough, moreover, an *ad hoc* meaning for *John laughed the soup on the table* can be derived by imbuing *laugh* with some of the semantic content suggested by its new syntactic properties, i.e., that the meaning is 'put, in a laughing fashion.'

The thrust of the preceding remarks is that the construal of various predicates restricts the surface structures in which they appear. As this begins to imply, the varying subcategorization frames in which a single predicate is used modify its construal. Consider the following examples:

(1) North Korea is similar to China.
(2) China is similar to North Korea.
(3) China and North Korea are similar to each other.
(4) China and North Korea are similar.
(5) North Korea and China are similar.

Tversky (1977; Tversky and Gati, 1978) showed experimentally that subjects' judgments of degree of similarity varied systematically for sentences such as (1) and (2): that *similarity* was interpreted asymmetrically in these environments. Though apparently the experimental test was not performed, Tversky assumed, and so do we, that (3)–(5) would not yield these asymmetric judgments. Thus the same predicate, *similar*, has two different, though related, interpretations marked in the surface structure, one nondirectional and symmetric, the other directional and asymmetric (roughly 'degree of match to some standard'). This dependence of construal on the syntactic environment is not an isolated fact about the predicate *similar* but rather is a systematic (though very complex) aspect of the fine structure of language design (see Talmy, 1983, and note 3 to this chapter for fuller discussion of these phenomena and an analysis of *similar* and related predicates). At bottom, this is why our position will be that the child learner can derive information about the predicate meaning by inspecting the syntactic structures in which it is embedded.

The relations between syntactic formats and the meanings conveyed by their predicates are by no means always as straightforward as they seem to be in the cases just discussed (*laugh, put, similar*). But there is no doubt at all that there are real and stable correlations between syntactic formats and aspects of verb meaning. We now attempt to show the semantic analyses of surface syntax that could in principle support a learner's inductions of the meanings of *look* and *see* (leaving aside the more difficult question of whether Kelli in fact performed such an analysis). The analysis proceeds in a number of steps, each property of the surface form contributing its small bit to the individuation of verb meaning. No one of these properties taken alone is very informative just because the relations between meanings and surface forms are complex and indirect. Rather, the distinctive syntactic properties act conspiratorily to partition the set of verbs into fine, semantically coherent, classes. We suppose that these syntactic analyses are not conducted in isolation from extralinguistic cues, but that these two sources of information are used jointly. In particular, the spatial analysis of the location of target objects (near, far, no object) provides crucial information for individuating the common verbs, but only if constrained by the subcategorization frame analysis.

Look *and* see *as motion verbs: Locative prepositions*

For the first step in the analysis, we follow a linguistic proposal by Gruber (1968). Gruber noted the rather surprising fact that the perceptual verbs behave syntactically much like verbs of physical motion, such as *fly* and *go*, in terms of the locative prepositional phrases they allow. We can say "John looked/saw over the edge of the cliff" just as we can say "John flew/went/wandered over the edge of the cliff." Most of the locative prepositions and adverbials can be used with each of these verbs: *up, down, behind you*, and so on. Kelli's mother freely used these locative prepositions with the motion verbs and a large subset of them with the visual verbs (Table 6.3). Table 2.1 shows that these locatives appeared very early in the speech of both Kelli and Carlo; Table 5.1 shows how they were used by Kelli in later spontaneous speech; and Experiment 3.1 demonstrates that Kelli comprehended the distinctions among the prepositions when they were used with *look*.

Gruber holds that notionally too the verbs of motion and exploratory perception are related: The meaning of *look* involves something like 'move the gaze to or toward' (or in Kelli's case, 'move the hand to or toward'). In general, Gruber's position is that this similarity in meaning is implicated in the similar syntactic behavior of these verbs. Verbs of motion will take locative prepositions and particles freely for semantically transparent reasons, and *look* and *see* will take these same prepositions and particles for the same reasons. (Of course, *look* and *see* are not merely motion verbs, but are special in encoding perception; we will take up their additional properties presently.)

If Kelli's interpretation of haptic exploration is motional, and if she was able to carry out the syntactic analysis of her mother's speech described in Table 6.3 (an analysis for the subcategorization frames of the common verbs), she would be in a position to make an initial partitioning of the set of verbs she commonly heard. The verbs *look, see, give, put, hold, come,* and *go* take locative-spatial prepositions, particles, and adverbials freely, but *have, play,* and *say* do not. Indeed one can say (something) *to* another, one can have something *in* hand, and one can play *somewhere* (in the garden), but the free use of the locatives—*up, down, in, around, behind you*—in prepositional phrases and as adverbial particles distinguishes the set of motion verbs from *have, play,* and *say,* which are highly restricted in the locative prepositions they allow (always excepting the idiomatic uses such as *have it out with someone, play up one's importance,* which do not appear in the maternal corpus). In this regard, *look* and *see* pattern together with the motion verbs.

As a first step, then, let us assume that Kelli exploited these differential patterns in her mother's utterances and thus could remove *have, play,* and *say* from the list of possible candidates for the meaning 'explore haptically.' To repeat, the grounds would be that 'explore haptically' is an idea involving motion and hence must be encoded by a verb that takes locative prepositions freely.[4]

Look *and* see *as inalienable acts: No three-term argument structures*

Certain of the verbs of motion (*look, see, come, go*) express inalienable acts (movements) of the agent or experiencer, while other verbs of motion (*put, give, hold, get*) express acts of an agent that affect the motion of another person or object. For example, in *John gives the ball to Mary,* John is the agent who causes it to be so that the ball moves to Mary: It is not John who moves. However, in *John looks at Mary,* nothing moves except John's gaze. The fact that an external object (the ball) is moved in the former case but not the latter has a simple reflex in syntactic form. The linguistic expression of the agent uses one NP position in the surface structure, usually the subject position, but two more argument positions are still required to express the verb logic: one to express the moved object (the ball) and the other to express the person or place to which it moves (Mary). An agent can *give a book to Mary* or *hold up a book to Mary* but no agent can *go a book to Mary* or *look a book to Mary* (as usual excepting such special and semantically distinctive cases as *I looked him in the eye, I saw him out of the room, I went the distance with him,* or *I looked the ball into my hands,* etc., which Kelli's mother never uttered to her child).[5] In contrast, for the perceptual verbs as well as *come* and *go,* the experiencer himself (or his gaze or hand) is the one who moves; he is the inalienable agent of the motion as well as being the moving object. Thus only two argument positions are required for such verbs. And as Table 6.3 shows, the inalienable verbs *come, go, look,* and *see* never take three-term argument structures.

In sum, the presence of an alienable agent (as revealed by three-argument syntactic structures) removes *give, put, get,* and *hold* as candidates for the inalienable construal 'explore haptically.'

The two criteria so far mentioned (free acceptance of locative prepositions, nonappearance in three-argument structures) taken together, leave only *come, go, look,* and *see* among the set of verbs frequently used to Kelli with their hats still in the ring for the desired construal 'explore haptically.'

Look *and* see *as perceptual verbs: Sentential complements*

Certain syntactic properties are especially informative for how Kelli could distinguish *look* and *see* (perceptual verbs of motion) from the verbs of physical motion. *See* occurred with sentential complements in the mother's speech to Kelli (Table 6.3). Notionally, it is clear why this should be: One can perceive events, but one cannot physically move events. You can *see if lunch is ready* and *see whether Granny is home,* but you cannot *go whether Granny is coming.* Sentential complements with *look* did not appear in the maternal corpus, possibly because of the limited sample of utterances (in principle one can say "Look at Sammy run" as well as "See Sammy run"), but a notionally related construction did occur. This is the use of *look* with the free relative *how* followed by an embedded sentence, e.g., *Look how I do it.* In contrast, with the verbs of physical motion one cannot say "Put it how you want it." Since *come* and *go* (the only candidates other than the perceptual verbs that have survived the prior criteria) cannot appear with sentential complements or *how* relatives, only *look* and *see* remain as candidates for the construals 'explore haptically' and 'perceive haptically.'[6]

The direction of motion: Source, path, and goal

By hypothesis, the learner now has sufficient information to distinguish *look* and *see* as the perceptual verbs. The spatial analysis of Chapter 6 (near, far, no object), describing the extralinguistic contexts in which the verbs were uttered, provides crucial supportive information for distinguishing among the verbs of motion. Specifically, the verbs *get, come,* and *go* were often said when the target object was far or when there was no object (Table 6.2). Semantically it is easy to see why: The source position of the object of *give* is at the agent (the one who gives) while the source position of the object of *get* is away from the agent (John gives what he has but gets what he doesn't have, as action begins). In contrast, the inalienable mover in *come* and *go* can move either to or from some initial location, so we can say both "come/go away from" and "come/go to or toward." Thus the extralinguistic positional facts should be variable for these latter verbs, as Table 6.2 shows they indeed are, and the prepositional choices (*to, from*) vary accordingly.

Summarizing the facts here for the verbs of physical motion, *get* patterns with the extralinguistic situation "target object far from the agent of the action" and the prepositional choice *from; give* patterns with the extralinguistic situation "target object near the agent of the action" and the prepositional choice *to.* Joint consideration of the positional and syntactic facts, then, in principle allows the child to conclude that the indirect object of *give* is the argument representing the goal of the motion while the indirect object of *get* is the argument representing the source; and more generally, that *from* represents motion away from while *to* represents motion toward.

Now how do *look* and *see* behave in this regard? Recall that they often appeared in syntactic formats quite different from the one now being discussed (e.g., appearance with sentential complements), and therefore did not fare too well on the constructionally neutral analysis for location of the target object shown in Table 6.2. But in Table 6.4 the syntactic formats were taken into account, by showing the conformity of *look* and *see* to the spatial-locational predictions for selected syntactic formats only (*look at NP, look D, see NP,* and the interjective deictic formats). In these formats, we agree with Gruber that *look* and *see* encode motion, in fact motion that is source-to-goal rather than goal-to-source. Thus like *give, put,* and *hold*—and unlike *get*—their uses by the mother should in these circumstances fall into the "near" coding category, as Table 6.4 shows that they do in the preponderance of instances. In contrast, the two other verbs not yet differentiated from *look* and *see*, namely, *come* and *go*, pattern differently in their "near" proportion of use.

One apparent exception to this rule ends by strengthening the same point: With modifying *come* or *go* (*Come look at the cat*), the required position of the mover as action begins is controlled by the rules for *come/go*, while the direction or goal of motion is still controlled by the main verb *look* (hence the motional description of *come look*, though different from *look*, is still distinct from that of *get*). Accordingly, as Table 6.4 shows, the target object falls into the "far" category for such usages.

In sum, verbs of motion encode the source, direction, and goal of motion in special ways, marked by differential choice of argument positions and locative-spatial prepositions and consistent with the fact that the target object may (*look* or *give*) or may not (*get* or *come*) be nearby as action begins. If the idea to be expressed is 'explore by hand' then the target object must be nearby as action begins. Therefore *come*, *go*, and *get*, which fail this criterion of nearby-ness and always (*get*) or often (*come*, *go*) appear with the prepositional choices *from* and *away from*, cannot encode 'explore haptically.' We conclude that a learner disposed to perform comparative analyses of the situations of use against selected properties of the syntactic form can individuate the motion verbs and determine which of them encode inalienable acts (or states, see below).[7]

Distinguishing look *from* see

So far we have not considered how Kelli distinguished between *look* and *see*. It was shown that in fact she made this distinction quite well: She could report when her mother was looking but not seeing (Experiment 5 of Chapter 4), and she used the interjective query "See?" and the interjective command "Look!" in her own spontaneous speech (Table 5.1).

A number of subtle syntactic distinctions mark the notional distinctions between these two verbs. We can document that Kelli had evidence for some but not all of these from our small sample of her mother's speech. Perhaps a more complete sample would have revealed that all the syntactic cues now to be described were exhibited in the utterances Kelli heard. It may also be that the whole spectrum of these distinctions is not necessary for learning. What we can do is to cite certain known distinguishing syntactic-semantic clues to these two verbs, and point out these cases where our sample shows these clues to have been available to Kelli (again, should she have been disposed to use them).

Look *is active and* see *is stative.* Certain verbs express activities (*look, touch, put, accuse*) while others express mental states (*see, know, think, suspect*). We have discussed this distinction when describing Kelli's own speech (Chapter 5). Reiterating this distinction, it is natural to command another to perform some activity ("Look!" or "Accuse John of treason!"), but it is unnatural and often incoherent to command another to be in some state of mind ("See!" or "Suspect John of treason!"). Hence imperatives are quite unnatural with stative verbs such as *see* and are absent from the corpus, but imperatives are natural with active verbs such as *look* and appear within this structure in the maternal speech sample (Table 6.3). In contrast, it is natural to inquire whether another is in some mental state, and hence the interjective "See?" does occur both in Kelli's and her mother's speech (Tables 5.1 and 6.3). We conclude that Kelli had a basis in the maternal speech forms for assigning *look* to the category of active verbs and *see* to the category of stative verbs.[8]

Further distinctions between *look* and *see* are made in normal English speech. However, our sample of maternal speech is inadequate to document whether these further distinctions were actually modelled by the mother. But they are worth stating here, for they begin to show the wealth of syntactic devices that are potentially available to learners who might be disposed to make use of them.

Look *is agentive and* see *is nonagentive.* According to Gruber (1968), "an agentive verb is one whose subject refers to an animate object which is thought of as the willful source or agent of the activity described in the sentence." That is, John is the agent of hitting in *John hits Mary* and the agent of looking in *John looks at Mary.* In both these cases, John is doing something rather than being in some state. As Gruber notes, there are a number of syntactic markings of these distinctions. For example, *What John did was to hit Bill* is acceptable, but **What John did was to know Bill* seems unacceptable. In this syntactic property, *look* acts like all other agentive verbs, and *see* acts like other nonagentive verbs (compare *What John did was to look at Bill* with **What John did was to see Bill*). Similarly, *in order to* (purpose) clauses are limited to the agentive verbs (compare *John looked into the room in order to learn who was there* and **John saw into the room in order to learn who was there*). Finally, manner adverbials are natural with agentives (*John looked through the glass carefully*) but not with nonagentives (**John saw through the glass carefully*).

Look *is motion toward and* see *is motion to.* Recall that in Gruber's analysis *look* and *see* are verbs of motion, and hence they accept many spatial-locative prepositions. Yet, as he also showed, there is an important distinction within the verbs of motion. Some, like *head* and *aim*, express motion in the direction of some goal (*toward*), e.g., one can *head for/toward the milk, aim at/toward the screen.* Other verbs, such as *fly*, can express both motion toward but also motion to that goal. For example, both *The bird flew toward the tree (in the direction of)* and *The bird flew to the tree* (as far as, or to the goal of) are natural. In contrast, *The bird headed for/toward the tree* and *The bird aimed toward/at the tree* are natural, but not **The bird aimed to the tree* or **The bird headed to the tree.* In short, while many motion verbs can express both the *to* and *toward* notions, some verbs are limited to one or the other type.

As Gruber pointed out, the motion verb *look* is a member of the *toward* group and is excluded from the *to* group: One can *look toward the tree* but not *look to the tree,* one can *look for the milk* but not *look to the milk.* Notionally, *see* differs from *look* in belonging to the *to* rather than the *toward* group of motion verbs. It expresses movement to a goal rather than movement in the direction of some goal: **John saw toward the house, *John saw for the milk, *John saw at the screen.*

Summarizing, another important notional distinction between *look* and *see* is the distinction between motion in the direction of a goal (*toward*) as opposed to motion to a goal (*to*). We cannot document that the mother's use of locative prepositions with *look* and *see* was broad enough to have provided this clue to Kelli (though perhaps it was, and the small sample does not reveal it). What is clear is that, in the long run, here is another semantically important distinction between these two verbs that receives a clear marking in the overt syntax of the language being learned. (There are further complications in the description of the locative preposition choices for *look* and *see* which Gruber analyzes very revealingly, but we reserve their discussion until later.)

Summary: Syntactic and situational individuation of the verbs

We have described a number of distinctions among verbs in their allowable subcategorization frames (essentially, in the particles and phrases that appear after the verb itself in the sentence structure). We claimed that these distinctions are useful for separating *look* and *see* from the other frequent verbs and for drawing generalizations about their meanings. This is because, or so we conjectured, the subcategorization frames are at least partly a function of the semantic properties of the verbs (for related statements of this general view, see Fillmore, 1968; Gruber, 1968; Vendler, 1972; Jackendoff, 1972, 1976, 1983; Talmy, 1983). In particular, the semantic-syntactic relations mentioned were as follows (see Figure 7.1 for a summary).

—The concepts *look* and *see* are spatial and encode the notions of location and motion. Therefore like other motion verbs, they should freely accept a variety of locative prepositions, and they do. This syntactic property excluded *have, play,* and *say* as candidates for the meaning 'explore haptically.'

—*Looking* and *seeing* as well as *coming* and *going* are inalienable, disallowing an external moving object and thus removing all three-argument terms from consideration (*give, put, hold, get*).

—The motion in *look* and *see* is of the sort initiated at the actor,

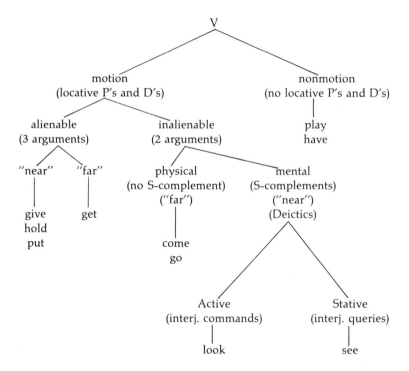

Figure 7.1 *A summary of the verb subcategorizations and situational contexts for the frequent verbs in the maternal corpus. For expositional purposes, this summary is presented in the form of a tree diagram, but it should not be read as a hierarchy. (The verbs are actually cross-classified rather than hierarchically arranged, i.e., it is not the case that the category "physical" dominates the category "active" or vice versa so far as we know.)*

and hence the particular choices of locative prepositions as well as conformance to the "far" category of the contextual analysis excluded *get, go,* and *come* as candidates for this construal.

—An important detail is that the use of *come* and *go* as auxiliary verbs modulates the encoding of source of the movement by the main verb.

—Perceptual as opposed to physical motion can be of an event, and hence only *see* appeared with sentential complements in the data base, and only *look* appeared with *how* free relatives.

—*See,* a mental state term, is distinguished from *look* in the corpus by disallowing imperative forms and allowing interjective queries.

Taking all these cross-cutting linguistic and contextual evidentiary sources together, it seems that *look* and *see* are the only candidates in the maternal corpus of frequent verbs for the desired meanings, if a learner is disposed to make use of such information. By hypothesis, Kelli was such a learner.

Learning Verbs by Recruiting Subcategorization Information

So far it has been asserted that syntactic patterning is probably a major evidentiary source for the discovery of word meaning. We argued that the learner is prepared to organize verb meanings in terms of a predicate-argument logic that varies over the verb set; that this logic is reflected in the subcategorization facts about the verbs; and that the learner has available, from sentential prosody, representational formats (surface parses) from which she can reconstruct these relations between sentential form and predicate meaning. We showed how the logic of the motion verbs, including the perceptual verbs *look* and *see,* is extractable—in principle—given these initial representations and biases.

However, we have given no specific account of how learning procedures that make use of this syntactic evidence might work. In order to do so, a necessary preliminary is to have a more global look at the representation of verbs in the mental lexicon. In this discussion, we shall bring in material concerning the adult lexicon that goes far beyond any accomplishments we have documented for the three-year-old Kelli—but it does describe the end state at which all normal learners, including Kelli, presumably arrive when language acquisition is complete. We first turn attention to two potential problems that any syntactically controlled model of verb learning must confront. Some of the syntactic frames for verbs may be arbitrary, language-specific, selections rather than necessary outcomes of semantic constraints on phrase structure. Moreover, since the mapping of meaning components onto surface forms is many-to-few, inferences from single verb frames to single meaning properties must be insecure. These very problems will begin to point the way toward a workable discovery procedure.

Arbitrariness and overgeneralization

There are difficulties for any learner inclined to take each surface property of the verb as providing secure information about its meaning. Untamed machinery that makes inductions from syntactic form to meaning or from meaning to syntactic form is fraught with problems. For example, it has been persuasively argued by Maratsos (1982) that it is dangerous in the extreme to conjecture that predicates similar in meaning (e.g., *like, fond of*) will share all syntactic environments; this would lead to the conjecture that *John is fonded of by Mary* is acceptable, by analogy to *John is liked by Mary*, or that *Tell me a story* would imply the acceptability of *Narrate me a story*. A few moments of thought, and the reader can come up with literally tens of such examples.

In sum, a learning device that required that all verbs with the same meaning have all and only the same subcategorization frames would be in an intolerable position, and would overgeneralize wildly. Such overgeneralizations do sometimes occur: A five-year-old of our acquaintance was heard to say "The people in this town wouldn't tolerate with that," presumably by overgeneralization from *put up with*, and a six-year-old wrote "The nice whale took everyone a ride," perhaps using the model for *give*. But as Maratsos (1982) has shown, such overgeneralizations are quite rare. The value of the syntactic analyses we have proposed, then, is limited by the apparent fact that some subcategorization facts are purely syntactic choices (which vary over languages, see Gentner, 1978, 1982; Talmy, 1983) and therefore are usable by the learner as clues to meaning only at his peril.

Thus there are great difficulties for machinery that seeks to draw simple generalizations about form/meaning relations, though many valiant attempts have been made. For example, quite a few investigators have suggested that there is a perfectly simple mapping between a small number of case labels and noun-phrase positions in sentences (Schlesinger, 1971; Braine and Hardy, 1982). In plainest terms, their work reflects the intuition that "do-ers of the action" are in English preponderantly subjects of the sentence, while "done-to's" are very often the objects; that is, that the relations between surface forms and their meanings can be stated by a few simple mapping rules. But a learner who believed in principle that such correlations were simple, and trustworthy over the predicates at large, would be quite misguided. It is enough to note that one can, meaning about the same thing, say either "That book collects dust" or "Dust collects on that book," or either "I fail to understand that point" or "That point escapes me," to realize that the relations of meaning to surface form, if real, must be extremely complex.

It is not hard to understand why the mapping between the surface syntactic verb frames and the verb meanings cannot be simple. As we have seen for some verbs known even to toddlers, a large number of semantic distinctions is encoded onto a limited number of phrase organizations of the clause. This many-to-few mapping of the meaning components onto the surface forms means that the child can make no sure induction from a single phrase structure to the meaning it encodes, or vice versa.

One might then suspect that learning verb meanings from their syntactic subcategorizations is a notion that is dead in the water. But we do not believe this is so. Though the relations between the forms and the meanings are complex, indirect, and imperfect, still—as we have tried to show for verbs such as *look* and *see*— there are many correlations of form to meaning that are very stable indeed. Charles Fillmore (1968) was the first to try to account for these syntactic-semantic correlations systematically within modern generative grammar, in a way that responds to the true complexity of language design. We believe that the approach now to be described is in the spirit of many of Fillmore's early ideas (though very different in the descriptive machinery envisaged; see Chomsky, 1972, for discussion of difficulties with the conceptual and technical machinery of "case grammar"). Clearly the present work is no place to present a formal linguistic mechanism for stating the syntactic-semantic relations—and no more are we in the most favorable position to devise the appropriate formal vehicle. Therefore the following discussion is perforce informal. In essence our position will be that the *set* of syntactic formats for a verb provides crucial cues to the verb meanings just because these formats are abstract surface reflexes of the meanings.

A conspiracy of surface forms

So far we have acknowledged that there is very little information in any single syntactic format that is attested for some verb, for that format serves many distinct uses. However, as we shall now try to show, the *set* of subcategorization frames associated with a verb is highly informative about the meaning it conveys. In fact, since the surface forms are the carriers of critical semantic information, the construal of verbs is partly indeterminant without the subcategorization information. Hence, in the end, a successful learning procedure for verb meaning must recruit information from inspection of the many grammatical formats in which each verb participates.

Relations between subcategorization frames and verb construals
It cannot be doubted that the same surface form can often be used for verbs that are very different in meaning. For example, the verbs *separate, steal,* and *take* can all appear in the same subcategorization frame

(6) NP_1 V NP_2 from NP_3

as in the sentences

(7) John separated the wheat from the chaff.
(8) John stole the candy from the baby.
(9) John took the trolley from Flatbush Avenue.

Yet these verbs seem to have nothing more in common notionally than the information encoded by the specification of the preposition *from* in (6).

Still the set of frames suitable for these three verbs differ overall. For example, *separate* but not *take* and *steal* appears in the frames

(10) NP_1 V NP_3 from NP_2
(11) NP_3 V from NP_2
(12) NP_2 and NP_3 V

as in

(13) John separated the chaff from the wheat.
(14) The chaff separated from the wheat.
(15) The wheat and the chaff separated (from each other).

More important, (11) and (12) are not just some more arbitrary syntactic frames that *separate* accepts. Rather, (14) and (15) are entailments of (13); for details, see note 3 to this chapter. In contrast, the entailments are not maintained between (8) and

(16) John stole the baby from the candy,

or between (9) and

(17) John took Flatbush Avenue from the trolley.

Moreover, *take* and *steal* sentences in frame (12) do not occur:

(18) *The candy and the baby stole.
(19) *The trolley and Flatbush Avenue took.

Two points are important from these examples. First, the sub-categorization frames allowable for a single verb are not independent of each other; rather, the frames are paraphrases of each other as in (7), (13), and

(20) John separated the wheat and the chaff,

or one is an entailment of the other, as in (14) and (13). Second, the allowable subcategorization frames, taken together, often tell a semantically quite transparent story, for they mark some of the logical properties of the verb in question. For example, the facts that *and* is substitutable for *from* (20 and 7) and that the order of NP_2 and NP_3 is interchangeable (7 and 13) have to do with the co-ordinate relation between NP_2 and NP_3 for *separate*. Moreover, the choice of the preposition *from* transparently marks the difference (direction away from rather than toward) between this verb and other symmetrical verbs such as *join* or *connect*.

There are verbs that overlap in many ways with *separate* in the sense just mentioned, but can never imply a symmetrical relation between the nonsubject arguments; this is marked by a fixed order of NP_2 and NP_3. Consider

(21) John tied Mary to the tree.
(22) John tied the tree to Mary.

In the former case, the tree is felt to be rooted in the ground and larger than Mary; in the latter, a small uprooted tree is the preferred reading.

These distinctions can be modelled in the subcategorization-frame specifications for each verb in the mental lexicon. A natural way to represent the fact that *separate* but not *tie* is a symmetrical verb is to enter a pair of frames for *separate*, differing only in the assignment of structural position for NP_2 and NP_3 (or else a lexical redundancy rule that generates one of these formats, given the other). In contrast, only a single frame would be entered for *tie*. This distinction models the fact that (21) and (22) are not paraphrases, but are just two different sentences using the same verb, just as

(23) Mary tied John to the tree.

is another one.

These examples, as well as the earlier analysis for *look* and *see*, bear on a more general point: The syntactic privileges of occurrence of verbs are intimately related to the concepts they encode. We have conjectured that significant aspects of the verb construals therefore can be extracted by the child learner from inspection of the set of subcategorization frames. However, the description of the verb lexicon just sketched is quite informal; and restricted in the items and properties considered. A more detailed analysis of the relational predicates such as *tie* and *match* is presented in note 3 to this chapter. This note reconsiders Tversky's analysis of *similar* by examining its behavior (and that of other predicates such as *kiss*, *collide*, and *argue*) under reciprocal conjunction. In our view, this class of verbs is particularly informative in revealing that the construal of a predicate is determinable only as it appears in specific syntactic structures. The further examples of *replace* and *substitute* are discussed in note 9. These verbs are of some interest to the present discussion because they differ considerably in their subcategorization frames and yet appear at first glance to be synonomous; just these examples have been used by Grimshaw (1983) to argue that relations between surface forms and verb meanings can be arbitrary, item-specific, language choices. Our discussion in the note is to the effect that these two verbs do differ in their construals, and in a way that is consistent with the differences in their subcategorization frames. A further example specially relevant for Kelli (the case of *look like*) is carried through in the next section; this example is used to flesh out the description of verb lexical entries that we have in mind.

But speaking here more generally, our suggestion is that it is converging syntactic clues for each verb, and their convergence with global information in the extralinguistic context, that turns the trick for the learners. It was a set of syntactic clues, not any one of them alone, which finally served to distinguish *look* and *see* from the other frequent verbs that Kelli heard (in the analysis of Chapter 6) and also to relate them to the verbs of physical motion (in the analysis given in the preceding section). Moreover, the extralinguistic environment (object nearby) was required to give a global clue to the gross semantic domain, to distinguish *look* and *see* from *come* and *go*. The same spatial analysis no doubt can be shown to distinguish Kelli's sense of *look* and *see* (perceptions that require proximity to the target object) from *listen* and *hear* (perceptions that can take place at a distance) and from *smell* and *taste*, which are not motional (note that one cannot *smell from here to there* or *taste at the cookie*).

The form of verb entries in the lexicon and the case of "look like"

The description of verb entries in the mental lexicon is taken to be in terms of such meaning components as we have just discussed: e.g., for the motion verbs, a description of the sources, goals, paths, directions, manners, and causes of these motions. In the scheme we have been developing, not all of this information is item-specific to individual verbs (though it is partly specific to an individual language design, a matter we will discuss later). Rather, it is our proposal that much of the information can be read off from the syntactic subcategorization frames themselves by a general scheme for interpreting these semantically. In English, part of this information is represented by the selection of the preposition (e.g., *to* rather than *from*), part by the number and placement of phrases marking the arguments. Thus we accept the orthodox position that each verb entry includes a set of subcategorization frames, but we add (perhaps more controversially) that these frames—necessary for describing individual verb syntax—do double duty: They represent part of the semantics of each verb.[10]

If this position can be defended, a necessary implication is that all the frames listed at a single lexical entry stand in an entailment relation to each other. For example, the item *report* would receive two separate entries in the mental lexicon, one corresponding to such interpretations as are intended when we speak of the report of a gun (an explosive noise) as against those altogether different interpretations intended when we speak of the report of a committee (a narration or account). Sometimes the choice between one and two entries for a verb is not easy to make (and might differ depending on the speaker). To see this point and to provide some detail for the general account, we now take up the specially relevant case of *look like* constructions, asking how they are to be represented in the lexicon.

A difficulty arises in proposing the entry or entries for *look*. Notice first that the machinery we have in mind does not require two verb entries for such sentences as

(24) John looked at Mary.
(25) John looked away from Mary.

One entry for the verb will suffice, even though these two sentences do not stand in entailment or paraphrastic relations to each other. This is because the distinct interpretations are fully predictable from the morphemic values of the preposition choices, making it unnecessary to state these alternate interpretations as properties of the predicate *look* itself. But the difference between *look at* and *look like* may be of another kind, a difference in the verb meaning (as was true for *report*). That is, *look at* means 'gaze at with the eyes,' but we have so far claimed that *look like* means 'resemble' or 'appear' (and hence behaved differently under the spatial-positional analysis of Chapter 6). But this could be the wrong solution, for 'inspection by eye' seems to be implied in both usages. Positing two independent lexical entries misses this fact, treating it as a coincidence.

It does seem possible to postulate a single entry for *look* by assigning the special construal for *look like* to a property of the morpheme *like*, not to the verb. Consider

(26) Arthur looks like a kangaroo (to Selma).

This seems to have a structure similar to

(27) Gleitman's textbook reads like a novel (to Selma).

Here the agent—often implicit—who looks/reads is Selma; the object looked at/read is Arthur/a textbook; and then *like a kangaroo* and *like a novel* have the construals they do ('as a kangaroo looks,' 'as a novel reads') in a way fully predictable by the item *like* and constructions in which it participates (along with other adverbial and adjectival phrases—*well*, as in *Arthur looks well* and *This novel reads well*, and *funny*, as in *Arthur looks funny*). If this is correct, then there is a single meaning of *look*, hence only a single entry for this item in the mental lexicon. Of course a construal rule of some complexity would be required to relate the surface form required in these cases (patient as subject NP, experiencer as indirect object NP, and so on) to the more familiar formats in which *look* participates.

Whether *look* in *look like* is to be represented as a separate lexical item (with the meaning 'resemble') or whether this meaning is to be derived from the ordinary sense of *look* plus *like* is not, however, a matter that can be decided simply by alluding to an analysis along the lines just presented, even if this analysis can be shown to work in detail. The real question is exactly how an individual speaker represents such items, and here it is possible that speakers differ.[11] Some individuals may represent *like* constructions in a systematic way over the set of verbs, allowing semantic reconstruction of the meaning 'resemble' or 'appear' for *look* whenever it is used with *like*. Other speakers may never have performed such an analysis and so may enter *look like* as a wholly distinct verb. Our interest is in a general scheme for the representation of verbs in the mental lexicon in a way true to whatever choices individuals may implicitly make. We hold that an appropriate device lists under a single entry a set of surface frames (or, where appropriate, redundancy rules that generate them) which stand in stateable paraphrastic or entailment relations to one another. Where such relations cannot be stated (as for *report*), two distinct entries are deposited in the mental lexicon. The extent to which formats are related differs in some degree for different speakers, and hence the number of entries they may have for a single phonological shape within a single lexical class may also vary. Particularly, where the construal rules are complex or else idiosyncratic to a very few items, learners may opt for entering the surface specifications as arbitrary, item-specific facts about the language.

The problem of conflation

The picture of verbs we have been proposing (following many authors such as Jackendoff and Gruber) is componential at heart. In the most general terms, the idea is that there are many semantic components that contribute to the overall meaning of a single verb, and that each (or, probably more correctly, most) of these components is marked syntactically and/or morphologically in constructions in which the verb appears. For example, the fact that *see* is perceptual is marked by its appearance with sentential complements; the fact that it is stative is marked by its nonappearance in imperative sentences and with the present progressive form. Taken together, we have supposed, these various morphological and syntactic features provide good clues to the components of the verb meaning.[12]

Yet it is not always the case that a particular subcomponent of a verb's meaning is marked by the surface forms of sentences in which it appears. On our story, any such defect in a verb's subcategorization frames should make its meaning more difficult for the child to attain, for we hold that the subcategorization frames are important clues to the meaning. To explain this problem, we begin by reconsidering the verb *see*. (Note that we continue to deal only with the core, modality-tied sense of *see* as our young subjects construe it, not with the extended or polysemous construals attained by adults, such as 'apprehend'.)

We have followed Gruber in describing *look* and *see* as verbs of motion. But as Gruber noticed, there is a single but clear-cut difficulty with that analysis. It was asserted that *see* and *look* differ on the *to/toward* dimension. Thus Gruber's analysis predicts that *see* should take the preposition *to* when encoding movement to the goal: The idea 'my gaze (or hand) goes to the top of the hill' should be expressed as *I saw to the top of the hill.* But notice that this sentence can be read only as 'movement (of gaze) *as far as* (the top of the hill)', never as 'movement (of gaze) *to the goal* (the top of the hill).' For the latter reading, English uses the form *I saw the top of the hill.* Gruber reconstructed an underlying *to* in the structure of such sentences, thus describing (though perhaps not explaining) this oddity in the syntactic behavior of *see*, granting its notional inclusion in the *to* grouping of verbs despite its unusual syntactic encoding. He claims, in brief, that a covert *to* appears in the underlying structure of the verb *see*, as shown in Figure 7.2.[13]

The idea here is that certain semantic properties (say the spatial-locative notion *to*) may be incorporated within the verb itself, rather than being exhibited in the surface structure with a separate lexical item. The arguments in favor of substructure thus become inferential, as opposed to claims made earlier based on observable distributional facts (the subcategorization frames). There is no evidence for a feature *to* in the lexical entry for *see* other than the construal itself—which is after all what is to be explained. Nonetheless, such covert elements are probably required in the description of verb meanings. Recall that we have already discussed a case (*nobody*) in which English conflates two quite distinct ideas (the idea of 'some indefinite person' and the idea 'negative') within a single formative—though in this case there is at least morphological evidence (the *no* in *nobody*) favoring the claim. We accept at least provisionally the notion that verbs may have semantic substructure not exhibited in the surface syntactic frame; in particular, with *see* the function usually handled with a separate preposition (*to*) is a component of the meaning of the verb itself.

As a simpler example of the same issue, consider the sentences *John comes into the room* and *John enters the room.* In the first sentence, the direction and goal of motion is expressed by a preposition and occurs cophrasally with the following NP (in the phrase *into* the room); in the second sentence, the direction and goal of the motion are exactly the same, as anyone who knows English understands without difficulty. But there is no preposition at all. How is the idea understood then? It must be that the verb *enter* itself incorporates the notion *to*—*to* occurs "in the verb," as a component of its sense, not in the following NP—and it occurs covertly: It is not physically marked by a surface linguistic formative.[14]

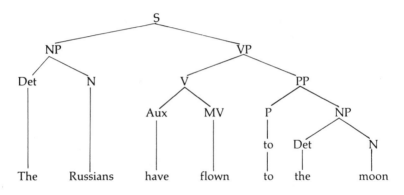

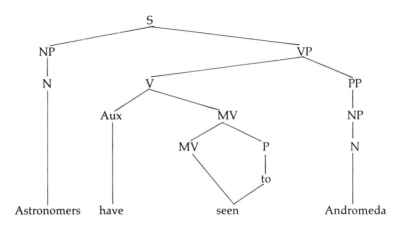

Figure 7.2 *Gruber's analysis of* see *(adapted from J. Gruber, 1968,* Language 43). *In this analysis,* to *is reconstructed in the lexical entry for* see *(see text for discussion).*

Let us now be frank about what this might do to the discovery procedure we have been considering. We have claimed that the surface syntactic properties of sentences, particularly the subcategorization frames for verbs, provide powerful clues to the meanings of those verbs. The missing *to* with *see* and the missing *into* with *enter* are among many examples that could be adduced to show that the correlation of syntactic forms with their semantic intents is by no means simple, direct, and inevitable. These examples pose no intractable problem to linguistic description, as Gruber among others has shown. But they do pose a difficulty for a learning device (e.g., Kelli) that is exposed to the surface forms and must reconstruct the meanings therefrom.

As Talmy (1983) has shown, these problems for discovering the logic of predicates from their subcategorization frames seem to be exacerbated as we look across languages, for certainly we wish the learning device to be as prepared to learn Ibo or French as English. If the surface markings for predicate logic vary wildly and arbitrarily across languages, the discovery problem for children— which semantic features to look for and how to expect them to be encoded—becomes intractable. But what Talmy has begun to show is that this general problem is not as devastating as might appear at first glance, simply because individual languages do not allow these conflations to occur arbitrarily. Instead there is a pattern of conflation characteristic of specific languages.

As one example, Talmy has examined the encoding of motion and location verbs in a variety of languages. Like Jackendoff and other authors we have mentioned (though with certain differences of detail), his analysis of the forms of motion verbs is componential, extracting a number of elementary meaning components such as 'path,' 'figure,' 'ground,' 'manner,' and 'cause.' He asks how these posited components map onto properties of the surface forms of predicates that encode them. For example, consider the notional distinctions 'motion' and 'location,' and 'manner' and 'cause,' as they appear in the following English sentences (from Talmy).

	manner	*cause*
motion	The pencil rolled off the table.	The pencil blew off the table.
location	The pencil lay on the table.	The pencil stuck on (to) the table.

In all four sentences (adopting Talmy's terminology), *the pencil* functions as the figure and *the table* functions as the ground. The verbs in the top row express motion, while those in the bottom row express location. The verbs in the left column express in addition a manner, while the verbs in the right column also express a cause. For each verb, the distinction *on/off* expresses the path.

A central question for Talmy (and us) is whether any and all such meaning properties can be conflated within verbs, or whether there are constraints on lexicalization (which meanings or meaning components can be regularly associated with the linguistic formative *morpheme:* in our case, with the lexical class *verb*). Talmy has shown that languages vary in the components they characteristically conflate within a single verb. As the examples just given show, English characteristically conflates manner (*roll*) and cause (*blow*) with motion and location. But even certain languages as close to English as Spanish characteristically disallow these particular conflations, requiring a separate marking for each component. Where English has *The craft floated on the water* (conflating manner with motion), Spanish would have to render this idea something like *The craft moved on the water, floating* (expressing the manner with a separate formative).

In contrast, Talmy asserts that English has only a very few verbs that conflate the motion and the figure (a counterexample is *spit*, which means 'for spit to move,' which is why *John spat over the side* is unambiguous while *John blew over the side* is ambiguous). But certain languages such as Atsugewi, according to Talmy, have scores of common verbs with meanings that show this conflation; he mentions as examples 'for a small spherical object (e.g., an eyeball, a hailstone) to move,' 'for a slimy lumpish object (a toad, a cow dropping) to move,' 'for loose dirt to move,' 'for runny icky material (manure, rotten tomatoes, guts, chewed gum) to move,' and 'for a limp linear object suspended by one end (a shirt on a clothesline, a hanging dead rabbit, a flaccid penis) to move.' These differing patterns of semantic conflation may provide a further clue to the young learner as to how to construct new verb lexical entries, given knowledge of only a few.

The syntactic means exploited to express the semantic components also vary across languages but again are reasonably consistent within a language, according to Talmy. To take one of his examples, in English both a verb "satellite" and a preposition are generally required to express the path: *John ran out* (satellite) *of* (preposition) *the house.* But in Atsugewi there is a set of satellites (appearing as verb suffixes), used without a preposition, which play these roles: for example, suffixes expressing 'into a liquid,' 'down into the ground,' or 'horizontally onto an object above the ground.'

Summarizing, languages vary in which meaning components are characteristically conflated within the verb, and in the surface syntactic or morphological resources for expressing these various meaning components. As Gentner (1982) has suggested, the differing conflation patterns must be learned, one reason why simple nouns (which encode about the same ideas in all languages) tend to appear before verbs in the child's lexicon. But the restricted conflation patterns aid the verb-learning procedure in the longer run by narrowing the hypothesis space: Though languages differ from one another, each language apparently is restricted in the choices taken. If so, the learner can depend on the notional conflations a language characteristically exhibits to guide inductions about the meanings of new verbs; and he can depend on the surface reflexes (satellites, prepositions, etc.) of the verbs to determine just how these notions will likely be mapped onto individual lexical entries.

The more general conclusion is that a verb-discovery procedure that is attentive to the surface reflexes of meaning components is not necessarily embarrassed by the finding that languages vary in what these surface properties look like. All that is required is that languages are narrow in their individual choices about how the meanings are encoded by the forms. Both English and Atsugewi (and other languages that Talmy has studied) appear to be selective and patterned in the way we would require if the learning device is to make educated inductions about semantic properties based on the spectrum of surface forms for individual verbs. What we *do* have to predict, however, is that occasional counterexamples to these language-specific patterns (such as the frequent absence of *into* with *enter*) would make certain verbs harder to learn than others—that *enter* will on average be learned later than *come in.*

Some Predictions about Verb Learning

We have proposed that the child has three major sources of evidence for the reconstruction of verb meanings: the conspiracy of surface formats, the language-specific patterning of verb-meaning components (and the syntactic resources for encoding them), and the inspection of extralinguistic context. It remains here to state explicitly why—beyond coverage of our own data—we believe a syntactically controlled procedure for acquiring verb meanings is a proposal worth serious consideration.

The all-or-none character of syntactic evidence

Syntactic analysis is an attractive hypothesis as an aid to the discovery of word meaning. One of its promising features is the potential for limiting the amount of data storage and manipulation required by learners.

The first economy has to do with *what* learners must store to acquire the sentential forms. In our view, they do not store heard sentences at all. Rather, the presumption with which we began was that even in early stages of the learning process the child can extract a phrasal parse of utterances from their prosodic properties, enough to individuate the semantically functioning phrases and to identify the verb. This parse of a heard utterance reveals to the learner a licensed subcategorization frame for the verb that appears in the utterance. If the learner hears another instance of the same verb in the same subcategorization frame, he stores nothing new, for no change in the grammar under construction is indicated by this further experience. Thus learners using this machinery must store only a limited set of abstract specifications associated with a verb, rather than the hundreds or thousands of heard sentences that may instantiate these specifications.

The second economy effected by a syntactically controlled acquisition machinery has to do with the reliability of the syntactic data base required for its construction: Syntactic information is essentially categorical. It is not as though "Go me to school on time" and similar monstrosities are rare events in the maternal corpus. They are virtually nonexistent (e.g., Newport, 1977, showed that there is only one dysfluency in every 1500 utterances from mothers to their young offspring). A learner who expects the information base to be this stable can, then, learn from only one or a very few examples in the corpus presented to his ear. He need not take into account the frequency of linguistic events, and hence he need not store or count huge numbers of instances (exactly the problem for distributional learning raised in Chapter 1). After all, in the end frequency has little or nothing to do with the question of what is grammatical: Less common passive-voice sentences are just as correct as active-voice sentences. As an example from the maternal corpus, progressive *looking* occurs only three times in the sample, but this may well be often enough for a learner who expects the input to consist of "good examples" only (and, of course, who is prepared to believe that statives cannot appear in progressive constructions).

In contrast, given the vagaries of event/word pairings (backs turned while hearing *see*, giraffes discussed outside the zoo), any machine that must map directly between the outside world and linguistic forms must be prepared to store and count many instances, perform arduous statistical analyses of preponderances, and the like. The daunting nature of this task is one good impetus for seeking alternative information in the categorical facts about syntactic structure. Another is the failure of the astructural Analysis 1 of Chapter 6 (Table 6.2) to describe what Kelli learned.

Waste not, want not: What is stored for the sake of learning forms part of the long-term knowledge base

Storage of event/utterance pairings is not only hard. Its value is restricted to the learning situation. Mature knowledge of English presumably does not include a summary description of how often or in what direction Mother crossed the room or what she was holding when an utterance of *give* occurred. That is, to the extent that such summary descriptions of events might be stored for the purpose of acquiring meanings, they are sure to be discarded when that learning is accomplished. In direct contrast, the subcategorization frames that we assume are stored in order to learn verb meanings are part of what constitutes language knowledge in the long run, and therefore are never discarded. The mature user must—forever—store the information that *give* has three arguments and thus can appear in such environments as *John gave the book to Mary* and *John gave Mary the book.* Otherwise she will never speak English correctly.

Thus the subcategorization-frame analysis has the advantage that the information storage it requires is known to take place and is implicated in mature performance. Each nonpathological speaker of English does acquire all this item-specific knowledge about the phrasal organization of the verbs, though it seems no mean trick to do so. If subcategorization frames are useful in explaining the learning, rather than being only the outcome of learning, the storage of all this information by the acquisition device is at least not wasteful or temporary. Rather, what must be *stored* on our hypothesis is exactly what must be *learned* to achieve mature competence in speaking and understanding.

The status of empirical evidence

There is some interesting descriptive and experimental evidence that gives initial support to the stance we are adopting. Carey's (1982) demonstration of "rapid mapping," the learning of new words from only a few introducing circumstances, suggests that the child is not dependent on repeated exposures to dissociating external circumstances for word learning, but is willing to make conjectures from a few positive instances.

Ninio and Bruner (1978) and Shipley, Kuhn, and Madden (1983) have inspected the syntactic-contextual supports in maternal speech for the learning of concrete nouns much in the way we have inspected the verb-learning environment, and with highly concordant results. Recall, for example, the discussion in Chapter

1 of the difficulties that attend learning even such a simple word as *rabbit*, and even in the favorable circumstances in which a rabbit is seen as the word is uttered: The child observing the rabbit observes also rabbit parts, rabbit properties, a particular rabbit, etc. Therefore, the question arises how, given the ostensive information only, one could learn that *rabbit* refers to the whole class of whole rabbits, rather than to a single individual (Peter Rabbit or Bugs Bunny), its parts (ear or mouth), or its properties (white or bobtailed). The investigators just cited have shown that relevant information exists in maternal speech. As one example, mothers when referring to animal parts will often (a) first name the whole animal and then (b) name the part using a genitive pronominal: "Here's the snake; these are his eyes." Particular rabbits referred to by name will have no determiner ("Peter Rabbit," but "*a* rabbit"). Rabbit properties are described by adjectives, a form class that patterns distinctively in the sentential parse. In short, form-class and syntactical distinctions can provide significant support for the rough guides provided by ostensive introduction of a noun or adjective.[15]

Prior evidence suggests a similar richness of syntactic distinctiveness in maternal speech within the verb domain. Notice that the syntactic learning hypothesis we are offering calls for complexity and variation in maternal choices among formats for an individual verb. This is because the verb meaning is not individuated in any one use, but by the spectrum of uses of that verb. Hence our conjecture is the opposite of the well-known "Motherese hypothesis" (cf., Snow, 1977; Furrow, Nelson, and Benedict, 1979). This latter hypothesis includes the idea that mothers will be restrictive in their choices of syntactic formats: They will say easiest ones first and then bring in harder formats when the child is observed to have learned the first (for discussion, see Gleitman, Newport, and Gleitman, 1984). But in our view, such a constriction can only delay the learner in finding out what the verb means. For example, *have* and *see* share some syntactic environments, namely V NP. We claim that if the overlap were complete, or complete at least as used by mothers of young learners, it would be materially harder for the children to distinguish among the verb meanings (indeed, if Gruber's analysis of *see*, as shown in Figure 2, is correct, the overlap is the consequence of a misleading encoding for that verb). So it is important to ask whether the required variation is really there in maternal speech. We have given some evidence that it is, by showing the spectrum of usages for *look* and *see* by the mother of even a very young and blind child

(Table 6.3). Thus the analysis of maternal speech, in which evidently no attempt is made by the mother to reserve a single form to a single function, is consistent with the requirement for learning if this is accomplished in part through the conspiracy of syntactic forms (for concordant evidence of form-function variability in maternal speech and gesture, see Shatz, 1982).

There is a small but interesting body of experimental evidence showing that such distributional information is recruited by child learners at least sometimes. For children as young as 17 months (Katz, Baker, and MacNamara, 1974) and also for older learners (Brown, 1957), it has been demonstrated that specifier choice (*a* versus *some* versus no specifier) affects children's hypotheses about whether a newly introduced term is a noun and, if so, whether a proper or common noun or a count or mass noun. That children recruit the available syntactic evidence for learning about word meaning to solve the wider variety of learning problems, and do so systematically over linguistic developmental time, would require extensive experimental manipulation to demonstrate (for an interesting discussion of the relevant issues and a lucid prospectus of the experimental programs required, see Carey, 1982). But we take the Brown and Katz et al. findings as at least initial support for such a program.

Though the studies so far cited are not inconsistent with our proposals, we acknowledge that they provide only indirect and inferential support. We do have pertinent experimental work underway, though it is at a very preliminary stage. Following a general line suggested by Carey (1982), we are attempting to teach new motion verbs to very young children in circumstances that seem natural (Gewirth, Gleitman, and Gleitman, in progress). The procedures involve introducing new verbs either as they appear in various syntactic frames (within brief stories), or by ostension (demonstrating, say, *rotate* while saying merely "This is rotating"), or by a combination of these two methods. Pilot results seem to indicate that (a) certain of the components of new motion verb meanings can be acquired by any of these methods by three- and four-year-olds, though there is an advantage favoring the ostensive and combined conditions, and (b) the relative utility of syntactic versus ostensive information is dependent in part on the particular verb to be learned and on the age of the learner.

We repeat that these are preliminary results, but they are much as we would have to predict on the basis of our hypotheses. Such verbs as *tickle* and *rotate* seem to encode salient and specific physical actions; perhaps ostensive introduction would be most valuable for verbs of this kind. In contrast, a more general motion verb such as *advance* is subject to a variety of construals ('move', 'move forward,' 'move to', 'move toward', 'push') when the learner is given a demonstration (ostensive definition). The various construals made available by ostension may be reined in, for example, by appearance of *advance* in the *toward* versus *to* grouping in heard utterances (John advances toward, not to, the tree), and its exclusion from use with *away* (one can push something away, but not advance it away).

Summarizing, some extant findings suggest that children can recruit syntactic information for word learning. Kelli's acquisition of the visual verbs suggests that she must have used syntactic information, for the situational evidence was sparse and at best probabilistically supportive for the inductions she made. Our own preliminary experiments begin to provide direct evidence that the syntactic context may indeed be recruited in the learning procedure used by children.

The underlying supposition of our analysis has been that syntactic support is required for verb learning owing to the apparent fact that the meaning of a verb is componential (consisting of such elements as motion, goal, path, cause). Since the components are differently conflated within different verbs in a language (*enter* versus *come in*) and across languages (English versus Spanish and Atsugewi), the process of learning comes down to extracting these components. This job is not easily done by parsing the world of events and scenes, as we argued in Chapter 6. But this parsing of the world is helpful if it is taken together with an analysis of sentential forms, for these are systematic—though complex—reflections of the individual meaning components of the verbs.

Despite what we think are enticing prospects, vastly more is left unknown than known from the analyses presented, even if they are correct in outline. We presented no proof that Kelli actually made use of the kinds of syntactic analysis we have proposed to learn the meanings of visual terms. It has been suggested only that such an analysis can work in principle. In reality, Kelli might have ignored all the syntactic information in her mother's speech and learned in some other way that we did not investigate. Perhaps she examined all the nouns that occurred with *look* as opposed to *hold* and was able to conclude that there was a systematic difference between "holdables" and "look-at-ables." Perhaps Kelli used some higher-level analysis of the event structure that we were not clever enough to discover and analyze. Despite these very real alternative accounts, the difficulty of bringing to ground a theory of learning that works simply by relying on "meaning in the world" suggests to us that linguistic-distributional analyses are worth careful pursuit.[16]

We note finally that a great deal of prior apparatus is required even if the present "syntactic support" argument turns out to be a major part of the true story of verb learning. The syntactic information described in this chapter can be of value only to an organism prepared to entertain the hypothesis that languages will formally encode the relation between motion and spatial-exploratory perception, the distinction between active and stative, and so on. That is, the distinction between concepts natural and unnatural to human learners cannot be dispensed with, but only enriched, by the information in the linguistic input.

Concluding Remarks

It has been argued that syntactic properties of verb forms provide a rich source of evidence for verb learning. At peril of belaboring what should be an obvious point, we dissociate ourselves from the implication that the forms of sentences transparently encode a small number of elementary perceptual and conceptual dimensions, reducing the problems involved in language learning to the discovery of a few simple mapping rules. The subtleties of semantic encoding even within simple sentences are too exquisite for any known machine, save human babies, to approach at all. The proposal we have given does bear resemblance to the proposals of Maratsos (1982) for a distributional discovery of lexical class assignment (for discovery of the partitioning of morphemes into verbs and nouns as opposed to the present procedure for making distinctions within the class of verbs). However, our proposal differs from Maratsos' on the important grounds that we suppose the linguistic basis for the child's discoveries is the parse tree, rather than a serially ordered string of morphemes (Gleitman and Wanner, 1982); moreover, we have here leaned more heavily than Maratsos on information extracted from the extralinguistic environment.

In sum, what has been proposed is a rather intricate distributional and contextual procedure for discovering the meanings and syntactic encodings of individual verbs. Even if it is correct in general outline, it is important to notice that only a restricted area of language learning can be so described. Any satisfactory theory of language and its learning must countenance a variety of contrivances and principles of organization that are far removed from matters semantic. Nonetheless, analysis of sentence forms against their semantic-structural content must hold part of the answer to how verb meanings are acquired. If this is so, perhaps it is possible to understand how Kelli constructed her systematic construals of *look* and *see* even though she was blind.

8 / A Blind Child's Understanding of Color Terms

> I think, it will be granted easily that, if a child
> were kept in a place where he never saw any
> other but black and white till he were a man, he
> would have no more ideas of scarlet or green,
> than he that from his childhood never tasted an
> oyster, or a pine-apple, has of those particular
> relishes.
>
> (John Locke, 1690, Book 2.I.6)

What can a blind child learn about a domain if that domain is forever and absolutely closed to her sensorium? The example taken up here has to do with color. Clearly Locke is correct in supposing that a blind child could never learn how to apply color terms correctly to perceived hues. Nevertheless, Kelli did learn something about color terms, a surprising finding if word learning is a relatively simple function of observations of the external world. The color terms are worth some discussion, given our overall interest in word learning, for a second reason. There is also a surprise about the way they are learned by *sighted* children, who can and do perceive hues: The color terms are notoriously hard to learn, are acquired relatively late in development, and with many errors along the way. Here and in Chapter 9 we raise the questions of how a blind child could have learned *anything* about color terms and why a sighted child should find their acquisition difficult at all.

The following examples (Bartlett, 1977) of two three-year-old sighted children's responses to the question "What color is this?" make it plain that they are quite confused about the reference of color words:

Stimulus	*Response*
brown shoes	S1: These colors are color shoes.
	S2: Shoes is color.

Stimulus	Response
pink watering can	S1: That color is thing gets water in it just like Mommy has. S2: You water it. Color is pink.
yellow chair	S1: That color is a chair, sit down, for sit down. S2: It's yellow.
green lamp	S1: That lamp is you turn on a light. S2: It's housey.

But as is also well known, these apparent confusions do not prevent many young children from using color terms all the same, at least to dress up their sentences. The two-year-old child of one of us, addicted to card playing, would set cards out in rows, saying "This is red one" or "This is blue one," though all were identical. According to Bartlett, appropriate matching of color names to hue experiences begins in the sighted child at about the age of three and a half. This is a good year after the appearance and appropriate use of many other adjectives such as *hot, dirty, big,* and *happy.*

Kelli, too, up until about age four, spontaneously used color terms and complied with requests to "Give me the green (object)," often saying "Here's the green one," without having any basis for doing so and of course getting the answer wrong. But from age 52 months, Kelli desisted from complying with requests to select or name things by their color and asked for aid: "Can you help me?" Thus in a period not too much later than sighted children map color words onto perceived hues, Kelli seemed to have learned that she had no basis for a mapping between these words and her perceptual world.

Kelli's Comprehension of Color Terms

In light of Kelli's spontaneous use of color terms, we tried to find out how she organized them and what she thought they meant, though the probes we conducted and the conclusions that can be drawn from them are much more limited than was the case for the visual verbs. A single experiment (Experiment 8.3) was conducted in the three-year-old period while Kelli still responded to color queries "as if" she could map them onto her sightless world. Thereafter, for some time we frankly failed to see the merit of testing her color use further. However, when Kelli was five years old, an experiment (8.1) was conducted to document that she had acquired a color-term vocabulary, and another experiment (8.2) was conducted to probe knowledge of an important semantic property of the color terms: that they pertain only to objects with spatiotemporal extent. These three experiments are presented below in the order that seems more useful for purposes of exposition, ignoring the real chronology. For Experiment 8.1, control data on sighted children are available from prior work by others; for Experiments 8.2 and 8.3, four sighted children close to Kelli's own age were also tested.

Experiment 8.1: What terms are color terms?

The question here is whether Kelli understood the color terms as a linguistically organized class of lexical items whose supernym was *color*. Essentially this same experiment has been conducted by Bartlett and Carey with sighted children (Bartlett, 1977; Carey and Bartlett, 1978; Carey, 1982), providing control data against which Kelli's performance can be compared.

Stimuli and procedure

At 60 months, Kelli was given a list of adjectives and asked whether or not they were color terms. The list was composed of sixteen color terms, six each of shape, size, and texture terms, and three each of taste/smell, sound, and abstract terms (e.g., *nice*). As a control for guessing, a subset of each of these terms was selected for their unfamiliarity to Kelli: four of the color terms (e.g., *indigo*, *puce*), two of the shape terms (*orbed, quadrate*), two of the size terms (*gross, minute*), and one each of the taste/smell, sound, and abstract terms (*pungent, shrill,* and *superior*). The set of 43 terms was randomized and presented to Kelli in the question, "Is ——— the name of a color, or is it not the name of a color?"

Results

As Table 8.1 indicates, Kelli knew which familiar terms are color terms and which are not. Her responses to the control words further indicated that she was not guessing. Thus while she had no perceptual basis for acquiring these terms, she at least learned a set of labels and their superordinate term. Notice that these vocabulary acquisitions present something of a conundrum for an acquisition theory that runs solely on the basis of meaningful interpretations of the *extralinguistic* contexts of use: Kelli learned ten words which in this case couldn't possibly be mapped onto the real world.

Table 8.1 *Experiment 1: What terms are color terms?*

	Kelli's response		
Perceptual dimension	**Yes, it's a color term**		**No, it's not a color term**
Color	black	pink	grey
	green	purple	violet
	yellow	white	crimson
	red	brown	indigo
	blue	orange	puce
			vermillion
Shape	(none)		round
			square
			triangular
			pointy
			orbed
			quadrate
Size	(none)		big
			little
			large
			small
			gross
			minute
Texture	(none)		soft
			hard
			scratchy
			smooth
			supple
			rigid
Taste/odor	(none)		sweet
			sour
			pungent
Sound	(none)		loud
			soft
			shrill
Abstract terms	(none)		nice
			good
			superior

Experiment 2: What can be colored?

We next asked whether Kelli's entry for color terms was semantically empty. For example, would she believe that ideas could be green? Though mindful of the difficulties of interpreting young children's responses to direct questions, we eventually began to ask Kelli directly what she knew about colored things. The primary question was whether she knew that colors can be predicated of objects but not of activities, events, or abstractions.

Subjects

Kelli was 66–72 months old when tested. Controls were four sighted children ranging from 54 to 66 months. The controls were chosen to be younger than Kelli based on our supposition—ungrounded, for the results presented here, as it turned out—that Kelli was maturationally younger than her chronological age-mates. She was still very small and had just been held back a year in school (repeating kindergarten) by directive of the school authorities. As will be shown, the upshot of this choice was that Kelli performed rather better than the sighted subjects (but not so much better as to make it worth running still more control subjects).

Method and materials

Following a procedure developed by Keil (1979), the experimenter asked the subject to judge and comment on a variety of predicates: "I'm going to say a sentence, and you tell me if it's OK to say or silly to say" or, alternatively, "Tell me if anybody could say it, or if it would be silly for someone to say."

Each sentence was of the form: "The *item* was *predicate*" or *"not predicate"* ("The story was talked about," "The flower was not alive"). There were eight predicates and each of their negations, falling into the following classes: *abstract* (talked about, thought about); *spatial* (over there, in the backyard); *perceptual* (heavy, some specified color); *animate-abstract* (alive, dead). These eight predicates and their eight negations were crossed by eight items, from four classes: *abstractions* (story, idea); *events* (the circus, a thunderstorm); *inanimates* (milk, car); and *living things* (dog, flower). Every combination of predicate and nominals, crossed by the negative of each, yielded a total of 128 queries. Since there were so many questions to ask, a number of testing sessions were required for each subject. The subjects seemed to find the task interesting enough to hold their attention over these sessions.

The sentences were presented in blocks, with two blocks of eight presented in each of eight sessions. Each block contained each of the eight nominals, presented with one predicate each. All predicates were assigned to each nominal in a randomized order that served as the basis for generating the blocks of eight. The first predicate for each nominal comprised the first block; the second predicate for each nominal comprised the second block, and so on. Justifications of the child's response were requested on a minimum of two trials per block. In addition, following the first two blocks, it became apparent that more justifications would be informative, and so from then all color queries were probed, as were all trials on which the child gave a nonadult judgment. Since the probes can introduce bias, it is worth stating in advance that requests for justification did not induce the children to change their original claim about whether the sentences were "good" or "silly."

Scoring

Responses were scored for two properties: (1) *violations* versus *nonviolations* of adults' judgments, for instance, if a child said that ideas could be green while adults deny the sense of this, the response was called a violation; and (2) *justifications* by the child were coded as to whether they made sense of the child's response. Within this category of "making sense" we allowed several kinds of response. The first had to do with a semantic or logical restriction on the use of terms (for example, a child responded "An idea can't be dead because it's really what you think about"). The second had to do with empirical truth ("The car was yellow because one of our neighbors might have a car that's yellow"). These two categories comprised the majority of both Kelli's and the sighted subjects' "sensible" justifications (.71 for Kelli, .91 for the sighted subjects—the sighted subjects being rather younger and thus opting for simple empirical truth more often than did Kelli). The remaining sensible justifications were either (1) when the child seemed to misunderstand by taking a word (here, *story*) that we intended in its abstract use and construing it concretely (here, as *book*): "The story was over there because they can be wherever they want but it couldn't stay outside . . . 'cause then it would get rained on if it rained"; or (2) where the child merely supplied a more appropriate predicate: "The flower wasn't heavy because it was really growing." Any response that didn't fall under these categories was called "other," for even if it made sense it was not the kind of sense we were looking for or could decipher. For example, we sometimes could not make head or tail of why the subject responded as she did, as in the following interchange:

E: "The thunderstorm was not heavy."
S: It's no good.
E: Why?
S: Because the rain, when you're at the circus, and then it won't be that much fun.

As can be seen from these examples, our results were not as coherent as those previously obtained by Keil. Still there was enough coherence to perform an analysis. Both 20 percent of the judgments and 20 percent of the justifications were independently recoded by a research assistant. The reliability of the two coders was .96 for the judgments and .82 for the justifications.

Results

Table 8.2 summarizes the findings. First, Kelli did not differ significantly from the other subjects in the extent of her disagreement with adult intuition about what can be predicated of terms (part A of the table). Though she looks slightly better than the controls for the color predicates in particular, the difference is not statistically significant (31 percent disagreement between Kelli and the adults, 52 percent disagreement between the control subjects and the adults).

Next the subjects' justifications were divided as to whether they had been scored as "sensible" (part B of the table). Kelli's percent sensible justifications for color predicates (.93) is not reliably different from the mean percent sensible justifications made by the sighted controls (.86). Similarly, Kelli's percent sensible justifications for noncolor predicates (.77) was approximately the same as for the sighted controls (.71).

Table 8.2 *Experiment 2: What can be colored?*

	Kelli	Sighted controls
A. Mean proportion of violations		
Color predicates[b]	.31	.52
Noncolor predicates	.37	.35
B. Mean proportion of justification types		
Total justifications[a]	.55	.78
Color predicates	.88	.97
Made sense	.93	.86
Did not make sense	.07	.14
Noncolor predicates	.50	.77
Made sense	.77	.71
Did not make sense	.23	.29

a. These include all justifications given by the subjects, either specifically requested by the experimenter or spontaneously offered by the subjects.
b. Though Kelli's color violations are fewer than sighted subjects[b], the difference is only of $n = 3$. Due to small total n of such questions, the difference between Kelli and sighted subjects is not reliable.

The central question concerns Kelli's (and the controls') justifications for the responses to color queries. Table 8.3 presents these in full for Kelli and a representative control. Inspection of the table reveals that with rare exceptions Kelli believed that objects, liquids, and animals can be colored, but that events and abstractions cannot. Her justifications sometimes were remarkably astute. For example, she said of the possible greenness of thunderstorms: "Really not any color . . . just out there roaring like a lion." (It may be important to recall here that Kelli was not linguistically precocious but fell in the bottom quartile of linguistic-developmental rate for blind youngsters). Though some of her justifications were not as close to the mark, some of those made by the sighted controls were at least as odd. Thus, in explaining why stories can't be green, a sighted subject reasoned "They don't have to be green if they don't want to." (Of course this response was coded as "other," i.e., not sensible).

For each concrete noun, Kelli judged that it could be some color. In contrast, there was only a single case where she seemed willing to grant that an event or abstraction could be any color at all ("green circuses," see Table 8.3), and maybe it was we who chose poor materials rather than the child who made a category error (it is too easy to construe this as the color of the tent, with the effect that two of the four sighted subjects also responded to

Table 8.3 *Justifications for color predicates*

Predicate and item	Judgments and justifications (+: it's okay; −: it's not okay)	
	Kelli	Sighted control
Idea—yellow	+ Really isn't yellow . . . really talked about . . . no color but we think about it in our mind.	+ Ideas can be yellow (but later, they're not any color)
Idea—not green	− It's to think about in your mind. (Could it be a color?) No.	+ Ideas can be green.
Story—green	− (no justification)	− (no justification)
Story—not green	− It's upstairs. (Could a story be green?) No. (Any other color?) No. (Could the *book* be any other color?) Green.	+ They don't have to be green if they don't want to.
Circus—red	− (no justification)	− (no justification)

Table 8.3 (*Cont.*)

Predicate and item	Judgments and justifications (+: it's okay; −: it's not okay)	
	Kelli	**Sighted control**
Circus—not green	+ It's really in Sommer's book. It isn't green . . . it's really someplace else. (Do you know what color?) White or blue or black.	+ Circuses are not green, they're usually yellow.
Thunderstorm—not green	+ Really not any color . . . just out there roaring like a lion.	+ Thunderstorms aren't not green.
Thunderstorm—yellow	+ Someone told me it before.	− They're a different color, sort of clear.
Milk—red	− It's really to drink. (Is it a color?) Brown. I don't know . . . raw milk.	− Milk is white.
Milk—not yellow	+ It's really at school . . . it's something else . . . it's a different color . . . it might be white.	+ Milk is white.
Car—green	+ Some cars *are* green . . . is your car green? (Yes) Good.	+ Cars are green sometimes.
Car—not blue	+ Our Toyota is blue . . . some cars are blue.	− We have a blue car.
Flower—green	+ Some flowers *are* green.	+ Flowers are green sometimes.
Flower —not green	+ It's really yellow.	− Sometimes flowers are green.
Dog—blue	+ A dog is not even blue. It's gold or brown or something else.	− Dogs aren't blue.
Dog—not green	+ Our dog isn't really green. Our dog is gold.	+ Dogs aren't green—I never see any dogs that are green.

Note: On another occasion, Kelli was asked, "Could a circus be (color)?" She responded, "Never been. We don't know what it looks like." Though the sample control subject does not justify as well as Kelli, overall the controls are not reliably worse than she. The slight difference is a consequence of their younger age.

circus as though it might be a colored thing). This distinctive pattern of responses to color queries about objects and nonobjects suggests that Kelli has some semantic knowledge of the color terms, enough to tell her that color is a property of concrete objects.

While the prohibition against colored events and abstractions was close to categorical, Kelli exhibited a lot of qualification and confusion about the color possibilities of *specific* concrete terms. This is not surprising. She receives occasional information to the effect that the dog at home is golden, the milk white, the grass green. As to the sensory basis for these attributions, she can have no clue of it. For her, color can be assigned only stipulatively. Hence she usually allowed that concrete objects can only be the colors she had heard them called.

But notice (Table 8.3) that for each object with extent Kelli believed it could be *some* color. Moreover, the justifications for rejection as between allegedly colored objects and allegedly colored events and abstractions were different. For the latter, she usually rejected all color terms and gave a different kind of justification. She usually remarked that such an event or abstraction could *in principle* not be colored ("It's no color, but we think about it in our mind"). In contrast, for sentences which used the wrong color label (green milk), she usually simply stated what the right color label was.

A similar response style characterized the sighted subjects. For the abstract terms, they usually rejected any choice of color, pointing out that these were "no color" or "you only think about it". Also, like Kelli, they rejected the idea that dogs could be green when they had no experience with beasts of that color; and in these cases they named the correct color.

Evidently the blind subject and the sighted subjects as well have a principled basis for predicating coloredness of some nominal terms and not others. Concrete objects are those that can be colored. Moreover, they realize that certain known objects that do partake of the property *color* are restricted as to which color. All the subjects quite reliably reject both green ideas and purple cows, but they know that the two phrases are problematic on different grounds.

Experiment 8.3: Nonvisual interpretations of color terms?

For the visual verbs as applied to sighted others (Chapter 4), we argued that Kelli could have made certain selected analogies from her knowledge of space and its labelling in her intact perceptual modalities. Thus hearing and touch might have been the source of her manifest understanding that some senses, including the sense of vision in others, operate at a distance and are differently affected by direction and barriers. Here we ask whether Kelli was ready to make analogies from her knowledge of a spatial property of objects (their size) onto a coherent interpretation of the color terms as used by sighted others.

This induction seems to have been available given the circumstances in which the mother used color terms to Kelli. These circumstances were quite limited because, not surprisingly, she found little occasion to use color terms to her blind child. Outside a single situation that we will describe, there were no uses of color terms in our sample corpus of 1640 maternal utterances (described in Chapter 6). Still we know the mother must have stipulated the colors of common objects on rare occasions, for Kelli did know that the grass was green, the dog golden, and so forth. To know this she must have been told. Why in these cases she bothered to learn what she was told, we cannot say.

In addition to these stipulative uses of color, there was a single situation in which Kelli heard color terms frequently as a three-year-old. In this one setting, she was potentially in a position to give color terms a regular (but wrong) interpretation onto the world of objects. She had a set of toy rings, each a different size, that were to be stacked on a rod in order of their size. This stacking game was one highly favored by Kelli, so she had extensive experience with this set of objects. Each ring was of a different color as well as of a different size (i.e., color name was uniformly predictable either from size or color). Kelli's mother habitually used the correct color term for each when showing Kelli how to use this toy: "No, you have to put the orange one on first." And Kelli correctly labelled the rings as she searched for them and manipulated them—"I need light blue one," "This the orange one," and so forth—showing that she did learn the labels corresponding to each ring color/size. Obviously her means for doing so was on the basis of size only.

By analogy with the results for the visual verbs, where Kelli commandeered a term from one modality (visual *look/see*) to her own operative modality (haptic *look/see*), we wondered if Kelli would appropriate the color terms for size or shape, given that the differentially sized rings could have provided her with an explicit basis for doing so. In essence, given that she had learned to associate a (relatively or absolutely) large ring with the term *orange* and a small ring with the term *blue*, etc., the question was whether she induced from this example the general idea that *orange* meant 'relatively or absolutely large' and that *blue* meant 'relatively or absolutely small.'

Stimuli and procedure

This experiment was conducted when Kelli was 43 months old: This is during the period when she was still willing to label an object for its color on request (recall that this kind of behavior, characteristic also of young sighted children, disappeared when Kelli reached 52 months of age). Four sighted children, blind-folded during the experiment, were also tested with the same materials.

The subject was given four sets of six kinds of object, each varying on a single nonvisual perceptual dimension but identical in every other way: six nesting cups of graduated sizes, three each of lucite squares and circles, three each of textured and smooth cubes, and three each of perfumed and non-perfumed cotton balls. She was presented with all items belonging to a set one at a time, randomized, in the following way. First her attention was drawn to the relevant perceptual dimension either by experimenter comment ("Here's a scratchy cube" versus "And here's a smooth cube") or by query ("And what shape is this one?"). She was then asked, "Please give this one to Mommy and tell her what color it is." In all cases, Kelli complied.

Results

Before presenting the results, it is important to notice that the experimental procedure itself reinforces a point that was documented before only with spontaneous speech data. In this experimental setting, Kelli showed no reluctance to respond with color names to color queries. In response to each query, she provided a color name.

Table 8.4 reports the color names supplied by Kelli for each of the six items within each category. The question is whether she transferred from the known uses of color terms as size markers in these new situations. As the table indicates, the size/color names of the stacking rings were not used as the basis for assigning color names to the nesting cups. Instead she guessed color names randomly with respect to the sizes of the cups. Moreover, some color names were repeated as the sizes of the cups changed.

For the shapes, textures, and scents, the same point is made in a different way. Kelli was offered, e.g., three indistinguishable rough blocks and three indistinguishable smooth blocks. If a color name were assigned on the basis of a physical property, the rough ones would get one consistent name and the smooth ones a differ-

Table 8.4 *Experiment 3: Nongeneralization of color terms to other known sensory-perceptual dimensions*

Stimuli	Guessed colors
Sizes	
stacking rings	red; orange; yellow; green; blue; purple[a]
nesting cups	blue; green; blue; purple; green; blue
Shapes	
squares	red; red; red
circles	black; black; red
Textures	
rough blocks	blue; green; blue
smooth blocks	blue; blue; green
Scents	
perfumed	purple; green; green
not perfumed	green; yellow; green

a. For rings and cups, the left to right order here corresponds to the size (largest to smallest) of the stimulus objects. Of course Kelli knew the color names for the stacking rings, so her selected color names for these were correct. She did not know the color names of any of the other objects, including the nesting cups, so for these she guessed a wrong color name except for a couple of random hits.

ent consistent name. But for six of the seven values of property types (the squares being a—presumably random—exception), Kelli changed color name within the same value of the same category.

The point of main interest is that, though Kelli heard color terms used directly as they mapped onto different sized and otherwise identical objects, and though she had acquired this discrimination for naming the graduated rings, she did *not* assume that the biggest member of any organized set of objects must be the orange one nor the purple one the smallest (as they were for rings). No more did she have *any* coherent strategy for naming the color of any new object, whatever its perceptual distinguishing traits.

As for the sighted subjects, three of the four could not be dissuaded from removing the goggles each time a color question was asked. The fourth subject behaved like Kelli. Since she had no basis for attributing color names when her eyes were covered, she guessed, thus providing one more instance of the finding that sighted children at age three are willing to use color terms without being able to match them against perceived properties (Bartlett, 1977).

Discussion

Kelli at three years of age did not form the induction, potentially available from the only frequent and organized setting in which she heard color terms used at that time, that these words encoded (relative or absolute) sizes of objects. It may be that this negative outcome requires no serious response. After all, there must be literally millions of situations in which children don't happen to attend very closely and therefore don't happen to learn very much. For the present case, the introducing circumstances involved only a single object type (the rings), perhaps too narrow a base on which to form an inductive generalization; moreover, there might have been such organized counterexamples as presentation of, say, two cups of a single size labelled with color terms (though no such examples appear in our sample of maternal speech).[1]

Nonetheless, Kelli's failure to form the size/color induction may be of some interest. After all, she did not forbear from acquiring the labels for color terms or from applying them to real-world objects. We shall return to this topic in Chapter 9, where we discuss "natural" lexical categories.

Syntactic Properties of Color Terms

We found that Kelli knew that ten color terms:

   —belong to a single domain whose supernym is *color*
   — are used in adjectival positions in sentences
   — can be applied only to concrete objects
   — do not map onto certain available perceptual property domains such as size, but rather
   — map onto a property that Kelli cannot figue out (and so she eventually asks for help in mapping that property onto specific objects)

There is some evidence from Marmor (1978) that older blind children may acquire even more detail about the semantics of color. Marmor tested congenitally blind twelve-year-olds, asking them to make similarity judgments for pairs of color terms. Their judgments in this task were coherent in preserving the warm/cool organization of these terms, though clearly they had no direct experience of the physical basis for these relations. (Work in progress from Park, Tsukagoshi, and Landau, which we will discuss in Chapter 9, suggests the same binary partitioning as a step in the acquisition of color terms by sighted three-year-olds).

How could blind children learn what they do about the color terms? Since relevant observations of the world are not available, there must be some other source of information. As before, we suggest that this alternate source of information is language itself. Much as was the case for verbs, there is syntactic organization in the color-term domain that may constitute support for blind children's limited but not insignificant learning.

Adjectives tend to encode properties

There is a strong though not perfect correlation between the lexical category *adjective* and the semantic category *property*. Some nouns do encode such properties as numerosity (a *lot*, a *bunch*, a *score*), shape (a *triangle*, a *circle*), and relationship (a *brother*, an *uncle*, a *friend*). Also, sometimes adjectives are used nominally to encode objects (The *rich* get richer, *Seven* came to dinner). But at least in the common vocabulary used by parents to their small children it is a pretty safe bet that a heard adjective encodes a perceptual (*small*, *rough*) or conceptual (*nice*, *young*) property of objects or persons. Kelli's mother used the color terms as both attributive ("the red ring") and predicate ("that ring is red") adjectives, providing a strong though not infallible hint that these are property terms rather than names of objects or persons.

Adjectival classes

Adjectives often fall into subsets with specific lexically labelled values (*green* or *small* or *angry*) and a superordinate label for the dimension,e.g., size (with such specific values as *big*, *small*, *tiny*), shape (with such specific values as *round*, *square*, *triangular*), texture (*smooth*, *rough*, *scratchy*), and mood (*angry*, *sad*, *happy*). Specific values can be queried in these domains either by use of the superordinate label—"What color is this?" "What shape is this?"— or by a designated term from the set—"How big is she?" "How red was her face?" (for discussions, see E. Clark, 1973; H. Clark, 1973). Such queries and their appropriate responses provide an evidentiary base for the construction of an adjectival subdomain. For example, in response to "What color is this?" it is incoherent to answer "two feet tall" or "foolish," but coherent to respond "red." Presumably, in addition to the fact that color terms often occur in unified ways in discourse—where conversation may center on, say, the colors or sizes or shapes of things and where these property names often occur in list structures—the question/answer contexts give evidence for a supernym (*color*) and its lexically stipulated values (*red*, *green*, but not *big*.)

*The adjective sets map onto restricted perceptual
and conceptual domains*

Kelli's experience with common adjectives (*rough, square, big*) provides a basis for her knowledge that some of them map onto concrete object terms only, while another set (*good, nice, happy*) is free of this restriction (see Keil, 1979, for a description of these restrictions on how predicates apply to terms; Carey, 1982, and forthcoming; and Shipley and Kuhn, 1983, for related discussion). For color, Kelli never (in our corpus) heard counterexamples such as *the square thunderstorm* or *the green idea* but only *the red ring* or *the round ball* (though she potentially could have heard some difficult counterexamples, for in adult discourse one may remark on *a blue mood, green with envy,* or *purple prose*). If conservative in learning strategy, Kelli might conjecture that the observed restriction for *square*, etc., holds for other adjectives unless counterexamples appear in the corpus. As an example of such a counterexample, expressions like *nice idea* certainly do occur in the simple sentences heard by young children. By hypothesis, data of this sort can convince a learner that adjectives such as *nice* represent abstract properties and thus occur as modifiers for abstract objects. But evidently color terms are hardly if at all uttered to young learners in such contexts. These restrictions on the applicability of color terms may account for Kelli's repeated denial that ideas, thunderstorms, and the like, could be any color.

Conclusions

Both Kelli and sighted children when young respond with color names to color queries and often use color terms spontaneously. But in so doing they are almost always incorrect. Some time between three and four years, on average, sighted children learn to match (discover the physical basis for specific color attribution). In fine symmetry, Kelli at four years stopped giving color names in response to color queries. Instead, she began to ask for aid, having presumably discovered that she has *no* basis for specific color attribution. We take the changes of behavior for both sighted children and Kelli, at approximately the same developmental moment, as interestingly alike. Nevertheless, the difference in the change that took place obviously instantiates Locke's reasoning that a blind man cannot know color as a sighted man can: The color discriminations that allow mapping onto the world of objects surely are available only through the eye.[2]

On the positive side, however, Kelli acquired some impressive information about color terms. She learned the supernym *color* and many members of the color-term set (Experiment 8.1). She learned the color names for various objects in her environment (Experiment 8.2). Moreover, she learned something quite general about what color can be predicated of. She knows that ideas cannot be green, but no more can they be red; abstractions and events in principle cannot be colored because, as she states, "You only think about them in your head" (Experiment 8.2). And she did not form a false generalization about how color terms map onto the real world, despite apparently misleading circumstances (Experiment 8.3).

Is it reasonable, then, to conclude that the blind knowledge of color terms is partial knowledge of the "meaning" of those terms? We believe the answer should be yes. Taking our results and those of Marmor together, it appears that the blind can come to understand that the color terms encode a unified perceptual dimension applying to all concrete objects; that certain particular objects have particular colors; and that the various hues encoded by the color terms are related to each other systematically.

At the same time, the semantic knowledge of blind individuals in this domain is likely to be restricted in many ways. For example, they might not know that the color terms label qualitative rather than quantitative distinctions (that the sensation red is different from green or blue in a way that cannot be described as a matter of more or less), that color perceptions involve the components of hue, brightness, and saturation, that there is a distinction between chromatic and achromatic colors, that there are significant context effects in color perception (that whites look whiter against a black background than they do against a grey background), and so forth. Finally, of course, beyond the stipulated color labels of certain known objects, the blind cannot match the color labels to objects in the world.

9 / Speculations on the Concept 'Natural Concept'

> Nobody joins the voice of a sheep with the shape of a horse, nor the color of lead with the weight and fixedness of gold, to be the complex ideas of any real substances; unless he has a mind to fill his head with chimeras, and his discourse with unintelligible words.
>
> (John Locke, 1690, Book 3.VI.28)

Our attempts to account for blind children's language learning have all been hedged about with an important proviso: The child learns words from the ambient linguistic and extralinguistic information offered, but only within the bounds of categories that are somehow "natural" or "salient." As one example, there is a problem in explaining why Kelli did not acquire the concept 'head tilt' despite explicit instruction and why the sighted learners did not acquire 'orient the head or face' as the meaning of *look* (for, after all, each act of exploring an object visually is also an act of orienting one's head toward that object). Now we attempt to come to grips with the problem of why 'head tilt' and the like are somehow less "natural" acquisitions than 'explore manually.' Thus we continue the long line of questions that began in Chapter 1 with rabbit parts and cats under mats, asking why such concepts are not learned even though they can in principle describe our transactions with the real world. It seems quite obvious that so long as this issue is left aside, progress in explaining the child's word learning must remain more apparent than real.

We need hardly apologize for the speculative nature of the account of this issue now to be presented, for understanding it is tantamount to understanding how an individual is inclined to parse his whole world. Therefore we shall not succeed in understanding it. What we will do is to examine some particular conjectures about natural lexical categories that our findings seem to bear upon. Beginning with the data from blind children and bringing in more findings concerning sighted children, South Sea Islanders, and other unlikely populations, we ask whether any sense or coherence can be made (at least by us) of the idea that some concepts are somehow more natural than others to express as words.

Limits of Learning from Experience

In essence, the work presented has asked how far the view of learning from experience can be pushed to account for just what is and is not acquired by the young child. Locke, as just cited, seems to have been optimistic, asserting that the concept 'baaing horse' is not constructed simply because no such creature is offered in human experience of the real world—but that such a concept *would* have been constructed just in case there *were* baaing horses. In short, he seems to have assumed that one learns what one experiences, little more, little less. It is from this perspective that the blind learners become an interesting test case, for their confrontation with the real world is different from that of sighted individuals and so ought to yield learning that is different in content. Indeed, Locke gave considerable attention to the blind on just these grounds (for example, in his consideration of Molyneux's question as to whether, if a blind man was suddenly made to see, he would upon first inspection recognize by eye the forms he had previously known only by touch).

Specifically, we have reported on investigations of four areas of the blind child's lexicon. These varied in how difficult they should be for her to acquire if it is true that learning is ultimately dependent upon specific sensory input. The first (Chapter 2) concerned the acquisition of the object vocabulary, for which blind learners seem to have an alternate sensory basis for environmental support. The second (Chapter 3) concerned the acquisition of *look* as Kelli used it of herself, again a case where she had alternate sensory input. The third (Chapter 4) concerned the acquisition of sighted verbs as these referred to the visual world and the visual experience of others, which she did not herself experience. Finally (Chapter 8) we studied the "pure" case of the color terms, for which the blind learner seemed to have no direct experiential basis at all. The findings are now reviewed to ask if the experiential facts are enough to understand what was and was not learned. Our own preliminary answer is "yes"—in fact, "of course"—but this answer is vacuous in the absence of analysis of the categories of experience which are natural to lexicalize. The bulk of what follows is therefore an attempt—however provisional and limited in scope—to come to grips with the idea of natural lexical categories.

Categories underlying lexical inductions: Vocabulary growth

At one extreme of the lexical domains we considered lie the items for which the child seems to be offered concrete exemplars in the world, words like *duck* or *spoon*. For these, both blind and sighted learners have relevant sensory information. Nevertheless, the exposure conditions of these children differ in at least two ways. First, the sensory experience of the blind learner is in the form of pressures on the skin, while to the sighted child it is in the form of sensations on the retina instead of or in addition to pressures on the skin. This may or may not matter (Locke would probably have voted no, but Berkeley certainly voted yes).[1] Second, even if equivalent information can in principle be derived from the differing sense organs, the opportunities to receive that information and the perceptual salience of such opportunities might still be different for those without vision. For instance, it was noted in Chapter 1 that visual stimulation is more likely to elicit systematic exploration early in life than is aural or haptic stimulation. Also, visual and haptic categorizations of experience seem to differ to some degree. (Recall, for example, Millar's [1978] finding that blind children exposed to braille dot patterns tend to generalize in terms of the density of the dots, while sighted but blindfolded controls generalize in terms of the overall spatial arrangement of the dots.)

Both these differences in the exposure conditions might lead to the prediction that the blind and sighted children will differ in their language growth patterns. However, as was shown in Chapter 2, the early vocabularies and syntactic growth of blind and sighted children were virtually the same. Moreover, the blind children's uses of their words were appropriate to the situations, so far as could be determined. Details of their vocabulary development closely mirrored that of sighted youngsters, bolstering the position that lexical concept attainment by the blind is quite normal.

Consider for comparison the data on sighted children. Gentner (1982) showed that normal learners in many different linguistic communities acquire nouns before verbs (object labels before action labels), and Bloom (1973) showed that they acquired object names before property names (*dog* before *big* or *green*). Nelson (1974) showed that they first acquire names for small moving things in their environment (*duck*) as opposed to large immobile things (*sofa*). Feldman, Goldin-Meadow, and Gleitman (1978) showed that isolated deaf children inventing their own gestured lexical items without formal linguistic input first devised manual equivalents for these same items. Mervis and Crisafi (1978) demonstrated that children acquire "basic level items" such as *duck* before superordinate terms (*animal*) and subordinate terms (*Chihuahua*).

All these generalizations about the course and content of the early vocabulary of sighted youngsters are true of the blind subjects as well. That is, they learned object names before activity and property names, terms for small moving things before large stable things, basic level terms before superordinates, and so forth, all in lockstep with their sighted peers.[2]

The findings of successful word learning by blind children are hard to explain if language learning truly requires specific sensory experiences, for these experiences were surely different for the two groups. The same findings will come as no surprise to many modern investigators who hold that the human representational vocabulary is at the level of perceptual, not "raw sensational" elements (cf. Hochberg, 1978), a position that presumably would predict the success of blind children with concrete object terms. Finally, as we have repeatedly stressed, these same findings *should* come as a surprise to clinicians who have assumed that blind children must be defective in learning owing to the specific sensory deprivation (and thus, for example, hold that the blind learner's use of *look* and *see* could not be meaningful, that it must be empty verbalism). After all, the expectation of deficit in this population makes sense only if learning words truly is a consequence of the specific sensory stimulation available to support it.

One might have supposed that modern students of language learning would not make the same predictions about blind children as the clinicians just cited. At least one might have expected them to be wary of making any predictions at all. This is because investigators in this tradition unblushingly traffic in such high-level descriptions of experiential categories as 'object,' 'basic-level object' (categories including *car* and *apple*, which surely are not simple sensational categories), 'property', 'agent of the action,' 'goal,' and the like. To the extent that language-learning investigators are unabashed in these terminological choices, it must be because they assume that (somehow) these categorial descriptions are primitive and thus *need* no internal analysis, for example, a sensory analysis of the kind offered by the British empiricists. But there is a paradox in the current literature, or so it seems to us.

The same authors who feel free to explain language learning by supposing that children "observe" objects, agents, patients, themes, and goals sometimes suggest that in principle a blind child's language learning must be abnormal all the same. For example, Fraiberg (1977) asserts that the object concepts of the blind are defective because of poor haptic-exploratory skills; Andersen et al. (1984) attribute the alleged defects to relative concreteness of representations; Bloom (1983) predicts langue use "disjoint in meaning" owing to the absence of "information from the context."

Summarizing, many investigators—correctly, in our view—accept categories that are remote from sensation as natively available to the human infant. Nowhere in this literature, to our knowledge, is it asserted that these abstract categories are shorthand labels for lists of sensory properties. These abstract categories are taken to be the primitive experiential bases on which language-learning inductions are performed. But, at the same time, these authors seem to back off from this set of assumptions whenever they are discussing the idea that language learning is based on extralinguistic context. In such discussions they proceed on the new assumption that the lack of *visual* experience must distort linguistic concept formation—that the peripheral input to perception significantly affects the character of the lexical concepts attained. Therefore they predict deficits in the blind population.

It seems to us that the descriptive facts about the blind subjects' vocabulary content and growth are a first indicant to the contrary; that, as Leibniz argued, "the geometries of the blind man and the paralytic must come together and agree though they share no images in common." That is, though the sensory sources of external experience may differ, this hardly matters, for the information from various sense modalities is evidently mapped in a sufficiently equivalent form onto central representations. If this is so, the blind may suffer no deprivation of relevant (perceptual) experience, thus accounting for why they learn the meanings of words "from experience" without apparent trouble. In sum, our findings concerning the vocabularies of young blind children are consistent with the majority of twentieth-century analyses of perception ranging all the way from Hochberg (1978) and the Gestalt psychologists to J. J. Gibson (1979). They are inconsistent only with a strict sensationist account. But such an account has no currency within the mainstream of modern theories of perception and perceptual learning. It only lives in a developmental literature which asserts that the blind have a defective context for learning language.[3]

A symptomatology for natural lexical categories

As an approach to understanding Kelli's (and indeed, all children's) acquisition of lexical items, we first draw on the idea that the would-be learners, while surely affected by experience, are heavily constrained by conditions on perceptual and conceptual naturalness. Such constraints have the effect of rescuing the learner's lexical inductive machinery from various pitfalls that experience places in its path: They must be invoked to explain why learners do not acquire absurd categories such as 'head tilt' *for which they do in fact have evidence.*

Jerry Fodor (1983) has suggested some provisional empirical symptoms by which to identify—though hardly explain—certain natural categories. In the discussion that follows, we will submit the findings for Kelli to some of these criteria, to see whether they can provide some rationale for what she did and did not learn about the meanings of words to which she was exposed. The relevant criteria are these:

1. Natural categories are among the earliest that normal children see fit to encode as words. The children derive these first lexical items from natural input (partly by ostension) without formal tutoring.
2. In contrast, other construals of these simple words, though made available by experience, are evidently never even considered by the young child.
3. Natural categories are lexicalized in the most common vocabularies of languages of the world, with only very rare exceptions.

We will try to show that Kelli's vocabulary items meet these initial criteria to different degrees, and that the circumstances and timing of their learning differed accordingly. We will also compare her learning against that of sighted children. To the extent that her learning accords in time and type to that of sighted youngsters, the blind child contributes evidence for yet another criterion of naturalness also put forward by Fodor, namely, that

4. Natural lexical concepts are learnable under widely varying contextual input circumstances: here, those of the blind child and those of the sighted child.

In sum, the first goal in this discussion is to point out that the lexical concepts acquired seem to have natural salience, and thus they emerge early and quite uniformly in the simple lexicons of natural languages, despite the varying circumstances of their users.

Look and see

As was shown in Chapter 3, both the blind and sighted subjects evidently learned a modality-specific construal for *look*. For Kelli the modality was haptic and for the sighted children it was visual. For all the subjects, the construal of the word was roughly 'explore, using the dominant modality.' A separate term, *touch*, was understood both by the blind and sighted subjects to mean 'contact manually,' a term much closer to sensation. Fodor's criteria for conceptual naturalness seem to be met for this aspect of the young child's lexicon:

Criterion 1: Early appearance. The perceptual terms *look* and *see* appear very early in development, before three years of age, in the vocabularies of both blind and sighted children. Kelli first uttered *see* at 29 months. From the beginning, most of her uses were as commands and requests to explore and perceive (though there were a couple of early uses as 'contact'). No attempt was made by the caretakers to instruct Kelli in this construal (see below). Thus *look* and *see* meet Fodor's first symptom of conceptual naturalness: early linguistic appearance, without formal tutoring. (The term *touch* was much rarer and later in appearance for Kelli. However, it was also rare in the speech of her mother, so nothing serious can be said about its timing relative to *look*.)

Criterion 2: Rejection of alternate construals. Availability cannot wholly account for what children first learn about the perceptual verbs. Alternative (sensory) 'orient the face toward' for sighted children, and 'touch' for Kelli were construals that would subsume the children's experience with these words, as we previously mentioned. Yet they did not acquire these meanings for *look* and *see*, as was shown in Chapter 3. In fact, as mentioned in Chapter 6, 'orient the face toward' was specifically modelled for Kelli by her parents in the context of a song-game, but this construal was not acquired even so. Similarly, neither Kelli nor the sighted children acquired the amodal sense of *look/see* ('perceive/apprehend,' where the source of the evidence in a particular sense organ is left aside) even though this interpretation logically must fit *more* of the maternal uses than the modality-tied construal—just because it is less specific—and indeed is a usage offered by Kelli's mother. Only this construal will really do for "Let's see if Granny's home," since it was uttered while the mother was picking up the telephone so as to ascertain—by ear—

whether Granny was home. Evidently 'perceive by use of the dominant exploratory sensory modality' is a highly accessible, natural interpretation, overwhelming alternates (some more superficial, like 'head tilt,' some more abstract, like 'perceive') that in fact are made available to the learner's observations of external circumstances. Thus the modality-tied construals of *look* and *see* meet Fodor's second symptom for conceptual naturalness.

Criterion 3: Lexicalization of look *and* see *in the languages of the world.* Fodor's third symptom is that the rock-bottom natural categories usually will be lexicalized—have single monomorphemic expression—with highly frequent items in the languages of the world. To the best of our knowledge, every human language has a simple word for the various modality-tied perceptual terms (such as the English statives *see* and *hear* and their paired actives *look* and *listen;* for discussion and evidence, see Joshi, 1975; Miller and Johnson-Laird, 1976). In contrast, terms for amodal perception tend to be rarer items (such as English *perceive, apprehend*) and are missing from the earliest vocabularies of learners. Thus the relative accessibility of the modal perceptual terms for novices (Criterion 1) seems to be mirrored in the facts about the vocabulary of the adult language: What is most "natural" is most simply encoded by the language.

Terms closer to sensation tend to be rarer. Often the language gets along without them. For example, English has no monomorphemic term for 'sensory contact with the eyes,' though in a restricted range it has a phrasal expression for this idea ("I never even *set eyes on* him"), or for 'nasal sensation' (excepting morphologically complex learned terms such as *olfaction*) as opposed to perceptual *smell*. More often, the perceptual terms are applied even when a low-level (contact) notion is implied by the context, as in these examples from Jackendoff (1983):

    (a) I must have looked at that a dozen times, but I never *saw* it.
    (b) I must have seen that a dozen times, but I never *noticed* it.

According to Jackendoff (see also Joshi, 1975), in "normal, stereotypical, veridical seeing" both conditions (fixing the gaze upon *x*, and having *x* come into one's visual awareness) are satisfied, and so by default a single term is usually sufficient. If not, special information is supplied as in sentence (b). In short, languages seem to have simple words for the modal perceptions, but are more spotty in an explicit sensory vocabulary.

This generalization is not entirely without exception. For example, English has a simple term for haptic sensation (*touch*) but seems to lack an adequate term for haptic exploration and perception. *Feel*, the closest candidate, does not seem to cover the range analogous to *look* very well. Indeed, it occurs only twice in the usage of Kelli's mother in our transcripts, suggesting that it does not adequately fulfill this role in everyday speech. But this gap in English appears to be accidental. Many languages do have a term for haptic exploration and a separate term for haptic sensation. An example is the French pair *toucher* ('contact manually') and *tâter* ('explore or apprehend manually'). Indeed, the French habitually use *tâter* to describe the blind person's manual exploration of the world. Thus Kelli's exploratory haptic term is not specific to her or to blind individuals in particular, but often appears as a common lexical item in natural languages. We suspect that had Kelli been learning French she would have acquired the two terms, *toucher* and *tâter*, rather than commandeering an item from vision (*voir*) for her haptic perceptions.

Summarizing, terms for modality-tied perception are among the most common verb items in most languages of the world. Modal terms for sensation are less frequent vocabulary items and often are missing. Specifically, a term for haptic exploration appears as a monomorphemic item in many languages (though not English), thus fulfilling Fodor's third empirical criterion for conceptual naturalness.

Criterion 4: Differing exposure conditions. The final relevant symptom of conceptual naturalness that we can discuss is learning despite differing exposure conditions. And our conclusion has been that Kelli, just like sighted children, can and did acquire the natural meaning of *look:* 'exploration, perception, by the dominant modality that discovers *objectness of.'* For this construal, she simply commandeered the visual-perceptual term. We suggest that humans, whatever their sensoria, require a term to describe their perceptual exploration of the world. As we remarked in Chapter 3, if like a bat some human child were sonar equipped, she might have chosen 'listen/hear' as the interpretation of /lʌk/ and /si/ given the same exposure conditions.

This essentially utilitarian description of the acquisition of haptic *look* leaves a good deal to the imagination. All we have said is that exploring organisms who use language ought to find it natural to encode these explorations early in life and by simple means—in the vocabulary of monomorphemic, frequently occurring words. And there is another problem: Kelli not only acquired a haptic interpretation of *look* and *see* (and *show*), but a visual interpretation as well. These construals refer to the exploratory perceptions of others, but not to Kelli's. We pause now to reconsider why these acquisitions seem to have been easy (and presumably natural) even so.

Clearly, Kelli had no visual experiences against which to match her caregivers' uses of *see* as it applied to themselves. Their *see* and her *see* do not compute the same relations to the world, for the visual terms apply to the activities of a distance receptor, one that is differently limited by barriers and by orientation of the body than the haptic terms. Our interpretation of this result was not that Kelli learned about the visual terms, visually interpreted, in the absence of experience. She has haptic-spatial information of the world she lives in. Her implicit but highly articulated knowledge of Euclidean-spatial properties of the world is materially the same as our own (as documented by Landau et al., 1981; 1984). And Chapter 4 showed that it was the spatial properties of visual *look* and *see* that Kelli abstracted: those having to do with distance, orientation, and barriers. Thus we conjectured that Kelli might have learned about the properties of sighted looking by analogy to the structure of her own sensory-perceptual experience.

But this account is insufficient. The explanatory problem for word learning is not resolved simply by pointing to the possibility of such analogies. The more difficult problem is to detail just how Kelli settled on these spatial features rather than on other available features of her experience to derive the visual construals. After all, there is no inevitable, direct, sensory experience to guide her: To acquire the correct construals, she must make just the right inferences, not many available wrong ones, from her derivative transactions with the sighted terms and the contexts of their use. For example, why didn't Kelli think that her parents' use of *see* (of themselves) was 'pretend to see' or 'hallucinate seeing' (say that you are—haptically—seeing even when you couldn't be, say, when you are at a distance from the object of inspection)?

The response to this problem made in Chapter 7 was that semantic-syntactic clues available from her caregivers' sentences (as used in apposite contexts) might have aided Kelli in singling out the right properties. It was argued that the syntactic contexts for *see* (use with sentential complements) imply that this verb encodes perception—just like *hear*, a verb that encodes the same perception for Kelli and her sighted caregivers. Verbs such as *pretend*, *dream*, and *lie* are associated with quite different syntactic patterns. Once this crucial hint has been culled from the syntactic contexts, the hypothesis that visual *see* is a term of perception is enhanced in likelihood. And since Kelli can perceive at a distance (by listening and hearing), so perhaps she can concede that if her parents claim to perceive at a distance and if *see* is known from syntactic evidence to encode a perception, this is likely true. They are probably seeing, rather than pretending to feel, when they say "I see."

Restating, part of the explanation of Kelli's learning of *see* is doubtless that her own sensorium of hearing, touching, and smelling makes available experiential analogies to visual seeing; these alternative experiences are probably necessary for the reconstruction of *see* by the blind. But these potential analogies are insufficient, for other, false, analogies could be made, e.g., to hallucinating or lying. We hold that the syntactic resemblance between *see* and *hear* (but not between *see* and *lie*) provides a crucial cue as to which analogy might be the right one.

If this approach is correct, it at last begins to provide some indication of why Kelli might have settled upon 'perceive *by hand*' (perception through use of a specific organ) rather than 'perceive' as her gloss for *see*. For at its most general the argument just given is that learners expect a certain parallelism among the lexical entries. As Shipley and Kuhn (1983) have suggested, learners expect the various items in a domain to be represented in about the same way. Children including Kelli presumably have evidence from their transactions with the world (conditions in which one can and cannot hear that implicate the ear; conditions in which one can and cannot smell that implicate the nose) sufficient to attach perceptual words to specific organs. If parallelism of lexical representation is a desideratum in constructing a lexicon, Kelli ought to expect *see*, too, to map onto the perceptions of a specific organ. The hand is her only choice.[4]

The larger point is that if Kelli has any problem at all in believing that her parents' seeing is like her own, she must share that problem with every sighted learner. A sighted child also frequently has the experience that her parents claim to see something and thus say "I see it" when the child observer himself cannot—as when a mother views an object from the near side of an occluding barrier and the child is at its far side. Still, it is apparently not so natural to conclude that the mother is confabulating or hallucinating when she says "I see it." Rather, her putative viewing is reconstructed—on our view, with syntactic support— by analogy to the geometric conditions of one's own viewing. The blind child's acquisitions from experience are hardly, if at all, more abstract than this.

Color terms

The case of the color terms lies at the far extreme of lexical domains we have considered, in trying to understand how word meanings are acquired from extralinguistic experience. Kelli could experience no colors. Nor does the haptic sensorium offer an alternative way of experiencing colors. In Locke's terminology, color is "of one sense only." Having the courage of his conviction that knowledge begins with and builds from sensory experience, Locke argued that the blind could never understand *red* or *green*. Indeed, as he (and of course everyone else) would have predicted, Kelli failed to learn to match colors to real-world properties of objects.

A first response to this outcome must be that this ought to be the end of the matter: Kelli did not experience colors and therefore did not learn to apply them to object properties correctly. What more is there to discuss? From our perspective, there is much more. Why did Kelli acquire the apparently nonmeaningful set of color terms at all, as Experiment 8.1 shows that she did? How did she know enough to limit their use to concrete objects, as shown in Experiment 8.2? And why didn't she transfer their use to apply to sizes of all objects, given that she discriminated among the ring sizes and identified each size with a ring color label (as described in Experiment 8.3)?

To approach the issues here, we first make a detour to ask about color-term learning in *sighted* children, again using Fodor's symptomatology for natural lexical concepts. This detour does not take us so far afield as might seem, because the blind child's failure to make the color-term-to-size induction may derive from the same cause that makes the color-term-to-hue induction difficult for sighted children.

Criterion 1: Late appearance of color terminology. As we mentioned in Chapter 8, sighted children often use color terms early in life, but they do so without being able to match these words against perceived hues. The recognition that color terms refer to hue categories is a relatively late acquisition. Astute observers have frequently noted this apparent oddity in lexical concept attainment. Charles Darwin (as cited in Bornstein, 1978) remarked upon it with some perplexity in his "Biographical Sketch of a Young Child":

> I carefully followed the mental development of my small children, and I was astonished to observe in two or, as I think, three of these children, soon after they had reached the age in which they knew the names of all the ordinary things, that they appeared to be entirely incapable of giving the right names to the colors of a color etching. They could not name the colors, although I tried repeatedly to teach them the names of the colors. I remember quite clearly to have stated that they are color blind. (*Kosmos*, 1877, I, 367–376)

Later, Darwin found that his children had normal color vision, and they finally acquired the color terminology.

What seems odd in the pattern of development is the difficulty of color naming in the presence of adequate color discrimination and even preference for unique colors over complex ones (that is, mixed hues) by the age of four months (as documented in Bornstein, 1975, 1978; Bornstein, Kessen, and Weiskopf, 1976). Moreover, it is known that young children find color an especially salient perceptual cue (Dodd and Lewis, 1969; Lewis and Baumel, 1970; Young-Browne, Rosenfeld, and Horowitz, 1977; and for a review, Bornstein, 1978), have extensive experience looking at colored things and hearing them named with color terms and frequently—as apparently was the case with Darwin's children, not to mention American preschoolers in Montessori schools—are formally "taught their colors." Even so, the pattern of color-term learning differs across children, is errorful, and often occupies a lengthy period of time (Carey, 1982).

Part of the lateness and confusion about color terms can be assigned to a wider generalization about lexical concept attainment. As we have remarked earlier, children acquire object names—"the names of ordinary things," in Darwin's locution—before property names (Brown, 1973). As a preliminary generalization, then, the relatively late appearance of property terms compared to object terms might suggest that the child is naturally prepared to encode experience in terms of whole objects, perceived qua objects (for a full account of this view, see Spelke, 1982; and E. J. Gibson and Spelke, 1983). As noted earlier, this pattern of development is hard to reconcile with Locke's derivation of knowledge from sensation (or, in modern guise, the hypothesis of "feature by feature" acquisition of nouns as described in E. Clark, 1973).

Yet the distinction just made, important as it is, insufficiently describes the special lateness of color-term knowledge. For both sighted children and Kelli, before the third birthday, have begun to use many other property terms appropriately. These include such size terms as *big* and *small*, locative terms such as *near* and *far*, rate terms such as *fast* and *slow*, and state terms such as *clean* and *dirty*, *hot* and *cold*. In contrast, appropriately used color terminology appears on average a year or more later in sighted children (Bartlett, 1977).

The difficulty of color-term acquisition has often been documented experimentally. Rice (1980) tried to teach *red* and *green* to children who knew no color terms (in the age range when some other children *do* know color terms). It took from 500 to 2000 trials distributed over two weeks to accomplish this! Thus Rice, like

Darwin, gives evidence for the special tutoring often required to inculcate the color lexicon. Also, children sometimes form an incorrect hypothesis about which color a term encodes, and such a false hypothesis may be very long-lived (Carey and Bartlett, 1978).

Carey (1982) discusses this range of findings with sensible perplexity based on her supposition that "the concept *color* is definitionally and developmentally primitive by anybody's account." We agree. But the fact is that color *terminology* is hard to acquire. The same children who readily discriminate and show preference among hues are failing to catch on to the reference of color-term vocabulary. Evidently the color terms are in some way relatively "unnatural."[5] Of course that unnaturalness cannot be perceptual. On the contrary, we have stated that children discriminate and show preference among hues even in infancy. Rather, the color terms seem to be difficult or relatively unnatural as lexical items, natural though it is to see in color. Thus they fail Fodor's first criterion for identifying the conceptual categories natural to encode lexically: early appearance without special tutoring.

Criterion 2: Rejection of alternative construals. In Chapter 8, we cited evidence from Bartlett (1977) that young learners often do not at first even construe the color terms as property terms, interpreting them instead as object terms ("These colors are color shoes") or function terms ("That color is a chair, sit down, for sit down"). Thus alternative construals available for the interpretation of color terms are sometimes chosen by the young learner, who later presumably revises them. Berlin and Kay's (1969) cross-linguistic evidence on the evolution of color terminology makes a related point. Many color terms are derived from object names: In Japanese the word for *brown* is *cha-iro*, with the literal meaning 'tea-colored'; French *cerise* ('cherry-colored') derives from the fruit name; many languages have a word for blood, which evolves toward the derived meaning *red*; and the English color word *salmon* is derived from the name of a fish. Of course we cannot prove that the evolutionary facts are different for adjectives such as *big* and *small*. Maybe once the first meant 'whale' and the second meant 'minnow.' But this seems most unlikely.

Criteron 3: Color terms in the languages of the world. Not only are many color terms derivative from earlier object terms. The color terminologies of the natural languages vary extensively in where they cut the visual spectrum (Berlin and Kay). The terms never violate the principles of color vision by establishing boundaries that do not respect the focal colors (the unique colors *red*, *blue*, *green*, and *yellow*, when these contain no admixture of other colors;

see Rosch, 1973, for the evidence). Quite the contrary, Kay and McDaniel (1978) report a rigid implicational structure for the terms that languages will encode. Nevertheless, the color terms differ greatly from language to language in other regards. Some languages encode only one contrast (which Berlin and Kay encoded as black/white, but which Kay and McDaniel revised as dark-cool/white-warm, based on Heider and Olivier's [1972] evidence from the Dani tribe's color terminology). If the language encodes three or four items, these will be those just mentioned, plus red-green. If it encodes five or six, yellow-blue will be added. And many languages, including English, encode many compound colors as well, such as orange.

Summarizing, languages differ in their color terminologies, though they are never incoherent with respect to the color spectrum. This lack of uniformity might be interpreted as an indicant that color is for some reason not a rockbottom basis for lexicalization even though, to be sure, it is a rockbottom category of visual perception.

Criterion 4: Different exposure conditions. Again we return to the blind child to see how these acquisitions take place under different exposure conditions. Kelli acquired some aspects of color terminology, despite her deprivations. She learned the set of color names and the restriction of their applicability to concrete objects (Experiments 8.1 and 8.2). But she obviously did not learn to match or to map the color terminology onto an alternative perceptual domain that was available, given her experiences (namely size, Experiment 8.3). The question is whether we can understand what Kelli did and did not learn about the color lexicon by further inquiry into the topic of natural property terms.

Relative and absolute property terms; two versus many terms

Four generalizations mentioned above require explanation: Color terms are learned late and with errors along the way; color terms are often misinterpreted by young children as object or function terms; languages always encode color but do so differently; Kelli acquired some, but not all, of the semantics of color terms. A distinction we believe is relevant has to do with whether property terms are *relative* or *absolute*.

The color terms are organized in terms of a range of absolute spectral values. The centers of these ranges are often focal colors whose perception is not arbitrary and which require no learning, but rather are given in the facts about the nervous system. That is, even though languages vary in the number of cuts they make in the visual spectrum, color terminology is not an arbitrary choice that languages make, but rather is coherent with respect to perception; particularly, one never has to "learn" to perceive pure red. But even though color terms map sensibly onto a nonarbitrary perceptual domain, they represent an organization that seems to be disfavored in *lexicalization:* Whatever the facts about hue perception, it seems to be the case that languages prefer to lexicalize relative property terms rather than absolute ones (Bierwisch, 1967; and see Talmy, 1983, for cross-linguistic evidence for this generalization). By the nature of the perceptions they describe, the color terms identify absolute (or close to absolute) cuts on a dimension. This may be one reason why they are hard to learn. Note again that what is hard cannot be making the requisite perceptual distinctions. The only thing that may be hard is getting the idea that there will be simple adjectives that represent these absolute ranges.

Consider, as another example, absolute terms for length, such as *inch, foot,* and *yard.* Here no nonarbitrary absolute values seem to be given by the perceptual apparatus. Though one can easily perceive the difference between an inch and a foot, insofar as one estimates lengths, the particular value *inch* has to be acquired by reference to some standard. Still such length terms are similar to the color terms in one way: They are absolute rather than relative. And just as for the terms of color, terms for absolute length differ across languages. A case in point was just mentioned: the American English terminology for lengths (*inch, foot, yard, mile*) as compared with the metric system used in England and elsewhere (*centimeter, meter, kilometer*). The variability of these absolute terms across languages is one of Fodor's symptoms for nonnaturalness of a lexical item. This fits with the fact that the absolute terms for length, like the absolute terms for color, are notoriously difficult and late to be learned, and show an errorful and lengthy period of development to get right.

There are also relative terms for lengths. These are much the same across languages (Talmy, 1983; see also Jakobson, 1939; Bierwisch, 1967; H. Clark, 1973). For example *big/small,* and *long/short* have simple monomorphemic lexical items in virtually all known languages. Moreover, they are apparently easier to learn than the absolute length terms, for they appear earlier than the latter in the vocabularies of young children.

Summarizing, we have noted two domains where there are absolute terms, one in which the values are perceptually nonarbitrary and one in which the values are arbitrary and must be acquired by learning. Despite this distinction, the absolute terminology in both domains is difficult to acquire and varies across languages. In contrast, relative terms in the same perceptual domains are easy to learn and seem to be much the same across languages. Our conjecture is that absolute property terms are less natural as lexical items and hence are harder for children to acquire than relative terms. We now will ask why this might be so.

Two facts about the absolute terms may be of importance in understanding their difficulty for learners. The first is the arbitrariness of the cuts they make in a dimension: What we call *miles* and what Englishmen call *kilometers* are different lengths, and where we have two color terms (*blue* and *green*), some other languages have a single term covering the whole range from blue through green. Surely the young learner, though he perceives that each of the focal colors is different, must remain openminded about where the language to which he is being exposed is going to make these cuts, just as he must remain openminded about the values assigned to absolute length terms in his language. The second problem with absolute terms is that if they are to map one-to-one onto perceptual distinctions, one would need very many of them. For example, humans can apparently make about seven million color discriminations and it is impractical for languages to encode these distinctions with seven million terms. The same is true, obviously, for lines of perceptibly differing lengths.

It seems that the common property terms that are easy to acquire and are the same across languages have to do with a relative binary contrast: *big/little, shallow/deep, fat/thin, slow/fast, high/low*, and so on. (Givón, 1970; Bolinger, 1977). What do these evidently more "natural" relative terms represent? They do not seem to represent the absolute top and bottom (positive and negative) poles on some dimension—*tall* does not mean 'tallest of all' or *fast* 'fastest of all.' Rather they refer to contrastive ranges, e.g., the range including relatively big things as contrasted to the range of relatively small things.[6]

Languages always seem to have such a polar pair for all the important perceptual dimensions. Further than this, no common lexical distinctions are made. There are no monomorphemic lexical terms for 'fairly close to the long side' or 'a little farther from the long side' etc., in any languages we know of. Rather, when a large number of such relative gradations are to be made, this is accomplished either by phrases or by use of a constructional lexical domain (morphologically complex, related items such as the English sequence *biggest, bigger, big, small, smaller, smallest*, or the Greek terms for temporal or spatial order, *ultimate, penultimate, antipenultimate*).[7]

We suggest that while children are perceptually prepared to

make a large number of absolute and relative discriminations among *properties* of concrete objects, they are biased toward the expectation that the common property *words* they encounter will encode relative rather than absolute distinctions. Moreover, their expectation is that this contrast will be binary; there will not be a large number of terms relevant to any single perceptual dimension.

The case for such restrictions on lexical encoding has been made most dramatically by Newport (1982, 1984) and Supalla (in press) in their investigations of the sign languages of the deaf. For the semantics of space and motion, concrete properties, and the like, American Sign Language (ASL) has available an iconic classifier morphology (though, to be sure, the iconicity is highly abstract). For instance, the term *walk* physically moves the hand whose shape represents the entity. The term *slow* is represented by moving the finger of one hand slowly along the other forearm. Relative size is indicated by a modulation of the hand shape representing the entity. Here the means are physically available for representing continuous gradations linguistically—either relative or absolute gradations: One could match the rates of movements in the signs to quite exact mimicking of the rates the entity is being said to move in. And memorization of a large number of distinctions would not be required, owing to the iconicity of the representations. Yet ASL does not encode these many discriminable differences either lexically or syntactically. It encodes two or three distinctions and no more. In short, even where the discriminations themselves are close to continuous and perceptually salient, and where the language has the formal resources for representing these many distinctions in a way that would not require enormous memorization, the language marks only a single binary contrast lexically. The provisional conclusion from the evidence presented is that lexicalization of relative binary contrasts is more natural or salient than lexicalization of absolute contrasts.

Kelli's acquisition of color terms

This much ground covered, we again return to Kelli. Recall that she potentially had a basis for mapping color terms onto absolute or relative sizes (the situation of the stacking rings). She clearly did learn such a mapping, for she was capable of giving each ring a distinct and correct color-term name; the basis must have been ring size since she could not see the ring colors. Still, Experiment 8.3 showed that Kelli did not transfer this mapping to new objects that differed in relative and absolute size.

Possibly this negative outcome can be assigned to the limited set of objects on which it was modelled (rings only) or—as we stated in Chapter 8—perhaps there were sufficient counterexamples (big brown cows, little brown jugs) in her experience to block this transfer. All the same, a striking fact about the acquisition of vocabulary in the normal case is the willingness of children to generalize their use of terms after a single or a very few exposures to one of their referents, as Carey (1982) has demonstrated experimentally. As she states, this willingness to leap to a lexical conclusion is documented not only in laboratory experiments but also by noting the sheer rate of lexical concept attainment during the first six years of life. Many thousands of words are acquired in these few years, the rate being somewhere between five and ten items per day.

Also it is extremely unlikely that Kelli received a large or systematic set of counterexamples to the potential size/color term mapping: Not surprisingly, considering that she was talking to a blind three-year-old, Kelli's mother provides no uses of a color word in the 1640-utterance sample outside the stacking-ring situation. So Kelli's failure to map color terms onto sizes may require an explanation that goes beyond the narrowness of the experiential base.

Preference for relative terms in lexical encoding. Our suggestion is that the difficulty for Kelli (in learning what, for her, could only be size terms) and the difficulty for sighted children (in learning color terms) has to do with the sheer number of the potential size terms presented. As Bartlett showed for color terms in sighted children and as was shown for Kelli in Experiment 8.1, the difficulty does not lie simply in acquiring ten or twelve separate phonological entities. This much all children seem to learn early and easily, consistent with their marvelous ability to acquire words rapidly and to store them just about forever. What is difficult to learn is not the items, but their construals. Our conjecture is that for the preferred relative contrasts, the child expects *an antonomous pair*, not ten or twelve terms: Kelli may have failed to acquire a (size) construal of color terms because there were so many of them that she never assumed that they encoded the preferred relative contrast (that is, the range from large to small). By age four, she simply asked sighted adults to tell her the colors of objects.

As for sighted children, they are bludgeoned at about the same late age to acquire specific names for certain of their hue experiences; formal instruction is usually required. But why do they find these difficult at all? Again, our suggestion is that the children assume that ten or twelve terms cannot be encoding a relative contrast, for the bias in lexical representation is in favor of binary specification of these relative contrasts.

These claims demand experimental demonstration, which we now have in progress. Most of the work is too preliminary for discussion here. But one procedure we have conducted (Park, Tsukogoshi, and Landau, in progress) both with Japanese and American preschoolers provides some weak initial evidence. The studies were conducted with three-year-old children who already knew the labels for focal colors in their language. They were shown 67 Munsell color chips and were asked to tell their colors. Indeed, the children called chips "red" that adults in their language community also called "red"—they gave focal-color chips their language-consensual labels. But what happened when the chip was of a nonfocal color? Here the children often erred, providing basic terms for nonfocal colors. But the wrong labels they provided were systematic. They never violated the warm/cool distinction: "Red" might be the response to an orange or a yellow but was never the response to green or blue. Apparently they honored a binary relative contrast (something like "relatively longer wave lengths versus relatively shorter wave lengths"). Related evidence for this same distinction comes from Isotomina (1963), who studied color naming and sorting in Russian children. She found that errors both in sorting color chips and in naming them preserved the warm/cool dimension. This was surely not because these children were perceptually juvenile and were inclined to see and notice fewer hue distinctions than adults or older children. Rather, on our view, language is expected to digitalize the domain in terms of a contrastive cut, though the perceptual facts about the dimension may involve thousands or millions of discriminable distinctions. Here warm/cool seems to be the natural choice.[8]

In sum, the problem in explaining the pattern of color-term learning is that it is perceptually natural to see in color, but the terms are hard to learn all the same. Thus while perceptual organization is doubtless implicated, by itself it provides too weak a set of constraints to account for the full patterns of lexical learning. The facts about exploratory perception were adduced to describe why 'perceive visually' was easy to learn without direct experience in preference to 'head tilt,' 'perceive,' or 'lie about seeing.' But the facts about color vision do not account for why learning hue terms should be hard.

So far we have assigned the difficulty of hue terminology to (1) the difficulty of property terms compared to concrete object terms, (2) the difficulty of absolute terms compared to relative terms, and (3) the preference for a binary contrast within the relative terms. Note then that on our account it is not anything about the complexity or substance of the hue—or form—domain that accounts for the word-learning difficulty. The problem for the word learners is not produced by the substance of these perceptual domains but by learners' expectations about the lexical encoding of these domains. Thus we have claimed that Kelli's failure to learn that *red* and *green* were size terms is the same as sighted children's difficulty in learning that *red* and *green* are hue terms.

Syntactic supports for binary splits. Syntactic distinctions between the relative/absolute split in property terms and the two/many distinction may ultimately be implicated in the patterns of acquisition. So far our story has been interpretable as a kind of disembodied "constraint" or "bias" in learning, one that favors relative binary contrasts over absolute multiple contrasts. But recall that in Chapter 7, the syntactic encoding machinery itself was asserted to play a causal role in learning: Verbs were said to be learned by a procedure that considers their subcategorization frames. Potential syntactic and morphological supports for adjectival learning were mentioned in Chapter 8. This latter ground is worth retraversing in the context of the present discussion.

We noted that the nature of adjectival domains is often cued in the questions asked about them and their appropriate responses, by superordinate noun labels: "What *color* is that?", "Red"; "What *size* is that?", "Two by four"; and "What *shape* is that?", "Triangular." For a certain subset of the property terms, namely the relative binary contrasts, it has frequently been noted that one adjectival—not nominal—term within the domain (*big* in the set *big/small*, *tall* in the set *tall/short*, and *clean* in the set *clean/dirty*) is picked out to serve this role in such questions as "How *tall* is he?", "How *clean* is he?", "How *big* is he?" *Big* is right in the question even if the "he" in question is very small. In contrast, "How *small* is he?" or "How *shallow* is the pool?" while not wrong are certainly infrequent and special in usage. (Notice, for example, that it is odder to ask "How small is that giant?" then "How big is that dwarf?") Thus there is often a polar adjectival pair, with one member selected to refer to the dimension without prejudice about the value on the dimenson (for discussion of these polar pairs with a so-called marked and unmarked member, see E. Clark, 1973; H. Clark, 1973; Carey, 1982). In contrast, though it is possible to ask of the absolute property terms—"How *red* is that?" "How *triangular* is that?"—these uses are comparatively rare.

It is clear, then, that a binary relative contrast not only is perceptually available but is syntactically identified in the language design. The dichotomy *big/little* is thus linguistically as well as ostensively made available to the learner. If that learner is, as we suppose, attentive to syntactic patterns, his learning of dichotomous adjective pairs ought to be facilitated: These are just the relative binary contrasts. As for further distinctions within an absolute adjective domain marked by a single nominal supernym (*color, length*), no further syntactic props seem to be available. The form to meaning pairing must be learned from extralinguistic context alone.

The thrust of our discussion has been that learning from extralinguistic context alone is difficult owing to the degenerate and probabilistic relations between scenes and utterances. How many properties special to some pair of overalls, in addition to their hue, could a child come up with as guesses for why his mother called them "blue"? They are also corduroy, dirty, small, two-legged, cozy, etc. Linguistic assistance, while it cannot erase this burden of hypotheses directly, can serve the function of highlighting the idea that a binary contrast is involved in the sought for construal. In sum, we believe that the unusual difficulty of acquiring the absolute property terms may be partly attributable to the linguistic nondifferentiation among them.[9]

Homonyms

We have subscribed to the very strong claim that there are constraints on what it is natural to lexicalize. In both the domains considered, we have suggested that perceptual constraints, though crucial, are too weak to explain the full patterns of lexical learning. For verbs, it was asserted that 'perceive' is no less perceptually sensible than 'perceive (manually or haptically),' and yet the modality-tied construals are uniformly learned before the amodal ones. For color adjectives, the ease of seeing in color did not explain why learning the labels turns out to be so hard. Therefore we added that further constraints exist for the word learner, the bias toward relative binary contrasts (which in turn may have its cause in its support in syntactic patterning).

But it is quite possible to reject the whole direction of our explanation, to deny that there are lexical constraints beyond those that are derivative from perception and human interaction. For instance, maybe 'perceive amodally,' 'head tilt,' and 'red' are merely ineffectual rather than odd or unnatural in some way. Perhaps the failure to learn them *in the presence of positive information* (exactly the same information that in fact leads to the acquisition of 'explore manually' or 'explore visually') does not require the assertion that there are natural and unnatural ways by which humans carve up their experiential world lexically. After all, it has often been argued that color is a superficial property that rarely classifies objects in a way that has utility: Whatever the color of the tiger, you'd better run. Better to concentrate on the size, the growl, the speed, the scowl.

But we believe there is a more general phenomenon that forces the conclusion that there are limits to the ways that language naturally parses our experiences of the world. This is the phenomenon of homonymity. Consider as an example the conditions for learning the word *dog*. Many different extensions (instances in the world that standardly fall under this lexical concept) are offered to the learner simultaneously with hearing that word, including the physically varying terriers, poodles, Chihuahuas, huskies, and Great Danes. Some of these exemplars are bigger than others, cuter than others, curlier than others. Some are potentially fearsome and some are not—while many of us are afraid of Dobermans, no one flees from a Pekinese. Yet despite these real distinctions, children readily assume that the single phonological object /dɔg/, heard in their presence, subsumes them all.

Now consider in contrast the conditions for learning the word(s) *bat*. Again, many varying extensions are offered to the learner simultaneously with hearing that word, including baseball bats and vampire bats. Yet no child, to our knowledge, assumes that there is a single category (perhaps, the prototypical flying black animal perched on a stick) that subsumes them all. Rather, in this case evidently two entries are deposited in the mental dictionary, available for inspection by the full panoply of techniques for testing "semantic memory." If it is doubted that children lay down two entries for *bat*, it cannot be understood how they come to laugh at puns.

Why is it that a single entry is sometimes constructed (as for /dɔg/) but sometimes two entries are constructed (as for /bæt/)? In both cases there is a single lexical entry offered, along with a varying set of exemplars. What explains the choice that learners make? It must be that there are natural perceptual and conceptual limits on the latitude of likely concepts. This supposition is not that the substance of lexical categories is totally fixed and cannot be stretched and reformed by the exigencies of experience, personal and cultural. One example will do to make this point. Consider the English lexical item that encodes 'little invisible electric balls that everything is made of and that, if you try to track them, go elsewhere.' Surely this concept (*electron*) is attainable and is lexicalized in the vocabulary of English. Still, at first inspection *electron* seems a less salient concept than *dog*. Though it is learnable, it is not easily and uniformly learned. As for the overall concept *bat*, subsuming certain mammals and sticks, it is never constructed even given a misleading linguistic code: The linguistic label for those mammals and those sticks is just the same one.

In sum, the existence of homonyms requires a perspective on language that is the reverse of the claim (cf. Whorf, 1956) that linguistic categories determine our modes of thought (though this claim might have some truth to it, it has been notoriously resistant to documentation). Homonymy, in contrast, is a widespread phenomenon in all languages, a fact so clear as to require no formal investigation. What it implies is that we carve nature in coherent ways to form lexical categories, no matter misleading information from the phonetic substance of those lexical entries, or from fallible and often confusing confrontations with the real world. The explanation at least in such cases as *bat/bat, trunk/trunk, bark/bark, no/know, homonyn/hominem,* and *common tern/Comintern* must be that no conceptually coherent idea subsumes the pair.[10]

We hasten to acknowledge that the real explanation of lexical concept attainment—or, much more likely, the set of real explanations—is clearly neither available nor even possible to guess at in the current state of cognitive developmental psychology. We have expressed the view that by and large it is investigators of perception who have made proposals relevant and specific enough to contribute to the issues here. However, a number of recent investigations have made a start, contributing detail concerning biases in lexical representation that go beyond the constraints established by perception. Examples include Markman and Hutchinson (1984) and Waxman and Gelman (1984). These authors have shown that young children tend to sort objects according to a thematic classification (told to "put the right things together," they group a dog with its bone rather than a dog with a cat). But when the children are given instructions that include a noun label ("This is a *snorg,* show me another *snorg*"), they tend to switch to a taxonomic classification. The implication here is that categorization performance in general differs from categorization performance as constrained by language. In a study we cited earlier, Shipley and Kuhn (1983) showed that the representation chosen for one class affects the representation of the next; the authors suggest that if, say, color and size have been specified in the lexical entry for the first bird name learned, then these same "features" will be specified for the next bird name, as if there must be some parallelism among the contents of various lexical entries. (See also Kemler, 1983, and Keil and Batterman, 1984, who have argued that the kind of representation changes over development—their view is that younger children tend to form "holistic" or "prototypical" categories while older children and adults tend to form "dimensional" or "definitional" categories.)

Such studies, like our own, try to ask how word learning is organized, since in principle the learner often has many choices among categorizations of objects, scenes, and events. Though current evidence on this general topic is fragmentary at best, such authors as just mentioned have begun to consider just what makes certain categorizations most natural under varying conditions. We have tried to offer one further detail to this emerging picture of systematic biases in the child learner which aid him in choosing among the lexical construals available, given extralinguistic context. We suggested that the learner has a preference for relative binary contrasts in adjective labels.

Our more general position is that an inquiry into the concept 'natural concept' is required if the topic of word learning is to achieve descriptive adequacy, or, indeed, any respectability at all. The fact is that nobody joins the voice of a sheep with the shape of a horse. More than three hundred years after the publication of Locke's *Essay*, we still don't know why.

10 / Final Thoughts

> Indeed the necessity of communication by language brings men to an agreement in the signification of common words within some tolerable latitude that may serve for ordinary conversation; and so a man cannot be supposed wholly ignorant of the ideas which are annexed to words by common use in a language familiar to him. But common use being but a very uncertain rule, which reduces itself at last to the ideas of particular men, proves often but a very variable standard.
>
> (John Locke, 1690, Book 3.XI,25)

This book has described an odyssey on which we embarked to discover how language develops in blind learners. Our underlying aims were not only to understand this special case, but more centrally to use the findings to reason back to the ordinary situation of sighted children acquiring their native tongue. We therefore close here by mentioning two interlocking paradoxes for understanding the construction of a mental lexicon by children, whatever their circumstances. Both are exemplified in the passage from Locke cited above. Since words are learned at least in part by inspection of their observed uses, and since each of us is privy to different observations, it could not be the case that all language users represent word meanings in exactly the same way. How does communication take place successfully if we severally mean different things by use of the same word? The second paradox is the obverse of the first: Language users do reach some tolerable degree of agreement about how words encode and describe the world. If the word meanings are straightforward derivatives of our varying experiences with their use, it certainly seems difficult to explain how we reach that agreement at all.

The Real Latitude of Word Meaning

Thus far, we have emphasized that there is a core of similarity to word meanings attained by Kelli and sighted individuals, and we attributed the similarity in what is learned to biases of perceptual, conceptual, and linguistic representation that override and repair certain expected effects of differing experience. But despite this real overlap, blind and sighted children do have different dominant modalities, eye and hand, through which they identify objects in the world. We would not wish to slide over differences in construal that this could lead to. Specifically, we glossed *look/see* as 'explore and perceive the objectness of by use of the dominant exploratory sense-modality,' and so claimed that the blind and the sighted children meant the same thing by these same words. But possibly we should have glossed these items by specifically referring to the appropriate sense modality ('by hand' for Kelli; 'by eye' for the sighted subjects). The findings presented in Chapters 3 and 4 demonstrate only that these terms as used by very young children are modality-tied. They do not directly show whether those modalities are named in the mental lexical entry.

Does anything hang on this? Surely it seems to. Throughout we have claimed that the blind and sighted children share the same entry for a term like *look*, but now it is acknowledged that they might have partly different entries for that term. If this is true, it suggests a revision of conclusions based on the same experimental evidence. In fact, it turns them on their head. On this new story, the conclusion is that blind and sighted children have partly different lexical entries for *look/see*—different in exactly the degree that is predicted by the difference in introducing circumstances. On this alternate hypothesis, the major problem becomes how to understand the success of communication between Kelli and her caregivers, now claimed to have distinct internal representations for the same phonological objects.

To examine this question, let us consider typical circumstances in which Kelli and her mother use the sight-related verbs. The mother might be holding a doll and will say to Kelli "Look at this doll." Whereupon the blind child walks up to the mother, takes the doll, manipulates it manually, and answers "I see." For some time, communication of this kind proceeds without obvious trouble, each conversational partner interpreting the item as suits her own perceptual life. Recognition that there is a partial mismatch of concepts in mind comes late and as something of a shock to both parties. Recall that the mother was astonished when Kelli responded differently when told to touch the doll (wherepon she tapped it) and when told to look at it (whereupon she explored it manually). The blind child, in turn, came late to the realization that her mother was using the sighted terms differently from herself.

The first such situation we observed was when Kelli's mother was showing family photographs to Sommer, her sighted child. Kelli was five years old, and Sommer was four. Kelli demanded to "see the pictures too," and the mother handed her what Kelli could only observe to be a number of identical flat papers. Kelli manifested considerable disturbance during this event, trying again and again to guess "who that is a picture of," and manipulating the photos by shaking, feeling, and mouthing them. After approximately fifteen minutes of failure, she asked, "Mommy, because my eyes don't work?" A few similar instances followed during this time period, for instance, Kelli's inability, in spite of stretching her arms, to be able to "see" a hot-air balloon passing over the car in which the family (and one of the experimenters) was driving. Her remarks (Chapter 5) that "You guys see with your eyes" and "I see with my hands" postdate these catastrophic events. But until this time, neither blind child nor sighted caregiver seems ever to have reflected that they were using the same words to encode partly different concepts. These new situations indicate the true state of affairs not because the internal representations are revealed to be different, but because for the first time those differing representations are shown to compute different mapping from the word to the world. One is sensitive to hue distinctions and brightness contrasts, and the other is not. Therefore to one observer the flat papers differ, and to the other observer they do not.

Partial differences among individuals in how they map concepts to words are all around us—they are hardly special to those with different sensoria. And, just as for the case of communication between blind and sighted, this hardly matters so long as the function from word to world picks out approximately the same objects, events, or scenes (Putnam, 1975; Kripke, 1977). Each of us can discuss iron with metallurgists and rabbits with biologists, despite extreme distinctions of what *iron* and *rabbit* must encode. Locke's example of these sure effects of different knowledge and experience on word meaning concerns a clockmaker and a clock watcher. He points out that the clockmaker "knows all the springs and wheels and other contrivances within of the famous clock at Strasbourg" and so must have an idea of it quite different "from that which a gazing countryman has of it, who barely sees the motion of the hand, and hears the clock strike, and observes only some of the outward appearances."

To correct for differences in the representation of words consequent on experience, and allow communication to go through, Locke suggests there must be tolerance for "latitude" in the word meanings, which are therefore "imperfect." But to the extent Locke is correct, one might wonder why we don't all mean wildly different things by all the words we are saying, resulting in such major breakdowns of communication as Alice observed in Wonderland. On a strictly empiricist story like that of Locke's, what keeps communication in hand is just that we are *not* in Wonderland. In our own land, nature so carves the world as to make certain inductions about the conceptual distinctions obvious to the point of irresistibility. As we have argued, however, such a position has trouble explaining why we do not encode the rabbits as undetached rabbit parts and acts of seeing as acts of orienting one's face (or hands).

Our position has been twofold. On the one hand, it certainly must be granted that the interpretation of a specific word must vary to some degree as a function of experience. Communication remains possible given this variation because it requires only that each of us has a mapping from word to world that picks out about the same things to be called by the same names. It does not require that each of us have precisely the same internal representation of the word or the same mapping rule. On the other hand, we have held that in this sea of variation there are significant islands of coherence and agreement across individuals, agreement that cannot be explained if external experience (which varies) is the sole determinant of the meanings of words.

To explain how lexical learning based on different introducing circumstances in some domains yields up categories whose substance and boundaries are much alike (e.g., *see* to blind and sighted children), we have argued that humans are endowed with richly specified perceptual and conceptual principles that highlight certain construals of experience and suppress others; endowed with linguistic principles about which discriminations among millions of salient ones are lexicalizable; endowed with principles for manipulating the speech presented to the ear in certain ways, but not in many other potentially available ways; and endowed with principles for pairing the perceptual-conceptual discriminanda with the lexical items.

The Blind Child's Problem
Is the Problem of any Learner

In Chapter 1, we emphasized special problems that the blind learner must confront, including difficulties in exploring certain large or distant objects manually and including special devices she might have to recruit to redress the imbalance of her experiences with those of her sighted caregivers. Yet the larger idea that our findings speak to is that the problem of learning a language may not be materially more strenuous for a blind child than for any other child, at least to the extent that learning *is* dependent upon extralinguistic experience. To see this point, consider another anecdote (this time one that is as much about ourselves as observers as it is about language learners).

Only one of us was present during the event of the photographs just described. The other observed only the videotape. On the small screen were two small girls with the same squeaky voices—Kelli and Sommer—engaged in a photo-identification session with their mother. The videotape observer who had not been present during the real event, having some trouble localizing the source of the speech from the tape, assumed that each childish query, such as "Which one is a picture of *me?*" was from Kelli. But this was false. Each of the two children from time to time expressed the same confusion of understanding. We tried to find out why by considering what the photographs portrayed.

The photographs were of the family's summer vacation, two years earlier when Sommer was an infant. Typical of the mother's descriptions was "And this is a picture of you" or "And here you're crying." What Sommer could observe was a silent infant in a crib, hardly Sommer's notion of Sommer. Such are the real conditions of language learning that obtain for both sighted and blind learners. Real-world contexts are provided, and these must provide clues that the child exploits to discover word meanings. But the situations are titanically more complex, various, and inexact as they relate to utterances than must be supposed by those who believe that word learning is "explained" by the assertion, true enough, that the speech of parents is accompanied by information about the world.

Notes

1. Language and Experience

1. The notation here adopted renders a number of distinctions we shall make throughout. An utterance of some word or sentence is rendered with double quotation marks ("dog"). Slash marks indicate that the phonetic description of that word or sentence is intended (/dɔg/), while single quotes represent the idea, notion, or meaning of that word or sentence ('dog'). We use italics to represent mention of the word or sentence, considered as an abstract linguistic formative (*dog*). Of course no special notation is employed where a word or sentence is used as a straightforward referring expression, i.e., when the word is used to refer to some or all extensions of the term. The standard notation is used when unattested or anomalous sentences are mentioned: They are preceded by an asterisk, e.g., *House the is red*, or by a question mark if their acceptability is doubtful. Our phonetic transcriptions follow Ladefoged (1975), except that we render reduced vowels with a schwa /ə/.

2. What is worse, in the account just given we have underestimated the problem of lexical concept acquisition by restricting attention only to certain "reasonable" options for interpretation that the learner might entertain. But it seems that in principle a number of "unreasonable" options exist if the learner is unwary. Such philosophers as Quine (1960) and Goodman (1966) have pointed out the scope of problems for a truly ignorant and openminded observer trying to learn concepts and words by inspecting the information available in the ambient environment. For example, on every occasion that an observer has positive evidence for having observed a cat (as someone points to a cat and says "cat"), he has just as good positive evidence that he has observed cat stages, or certain undetached parts of a cat or even something that is a cat until the year 2000, but will turn into a dog in the year 2001 (i.e., though observation may tell this learner that what is now visible is a cat, the observation itself says nothing about transformations this cat might undergo in future—maybe it will become a pillar of salt). There is always exactly as much positive evidence in the external world for each of these mad ideas as there is for the various nonabsurdities. But it is enough for us to con-

sider the reasonable alternatives left open by particular experience to understand the difficulties in making good the claim (doubtless true) that learning word meanings occurs at least in part by inspecting the real world.

3. This problem is worse if the learner assumes that English, like Latin, allows free positioning of the thematic roles. Some limited freedom in this regard does exist even in English: One can say "This book collects dust" and "Dust collects on these books" or "This garden swarms with bees" and "Bees are swarming in this garden" to mean closely related things. Thus even the child learning a word-order language cannot be too secure in supposing that a stipulated phrasal position in a sentence is a good guide to its thematic role. For further discussion of this point, see Chapter 7.

4. Examined more closely, Rosch's proposal here is not that the so-called basic categories themselves form the innate base for induction. Rather, such categories are taken by Rosch to have internal structure, in terms of some *other* vocabulary of simple (though not necessarily sensory) features: For the case of 'bird' these atomic features might be *feathers, wings,* and *beaks;* for the case of 'pencil' they might include functional features such as *for writing.* Presumably it is these features we have just called "atomic" that form the innate basis for induction in Rosch's view. On this story, what makes learning of the basic categories likely to the point of inevitability is that the atomic features are not randomly distributed over all objects in the world. Rather, "the structure of the world" is "correlated," in the sense that groups of features generally cooccur in certain creatures—and hence, according to Rosch, because we experience them together repeatedly, we associate them with each other, thus deriving such complex—but basic—categories as 'bird' (compare Locke, Book 3.IV.26–7, whose proposal differs only by the restriction of "simple ideas," or features, to the sensory ones). Clearly, then, the work of Rosch and others (see particularly Smith and Medin, 1981) continues the empiricist tradition in explaining language learning. Experience is in terms of a set of atomic categories (the features) far fewer in number than even the simple vocabulary items of a natural language. As for the basic level categories such as *bird* or *car,* if we read Rosch correctly she does not consider them to be developmental primitives but rather collections acquired by construction from lower level categories. In the literature, however, it is often assumed that Rosch must mean by "basic" categories those that are directly afforded by immediate experience. That may be the correct interpretation (one would have to ask Rosch or other proponents of this view) but in that case this position on lexical concept attainment would come rather close to Fodor's (1981). In fact, Fodor's own interpretation of basic level terms denies them substructure and takes them as the conceptual atoms underlying the lexicons of natural languages (see Chapter 9 for discussion).

5. Further observations by Fraiberg led her to extreme pessimism about blind children's prognosis for normal conceptual development. She argued that the spatial world of blind infants was virtually nonexis-

tent, that they lived in a spatial "void" that could be altered only by very active intervention with special clinical techniques. But many of the observations that led her to this view were of clinically deviant blind children who, for example, lacked functional use of their hands for purposes of exploration and object use.

2. The Development of Speech in Blind Children

1. Since this book was completed, we have had the opportunity to read an interesting new article by Mulford (in press). She culled from recent studies, by different investigators, information on language onset and early "semantic fields" in sixteen blind children; our data for Kelli, Carlo, and Angie are included. Her conclusion is that there is *no* onset delay (or abnormality in semantic fields) associated with blindness itself, for the sixteen subjects fell all over the normal range in moment of onset though clearly there is an effect of prematurity. In the whole group Mulford considered, Kelli and Carlo were among the latest to start talking, and they were the only premature births in the sample; this is consistent with the Norris normative results for a large population of blind premature children. If Mulford's sample is representative of the blind population, the findings reported in the text for our own subjects become even stronger. We will show normality in subsequent language development for even the premature blind subjects; given Mulford's findings, it becomes likely that this development does not even begin late (see also Bigelow, 1982). The relation between blindness and prematurity nevertheless deserves some further scrutiny. As stated in the text, our premature sighted subjects were delayed in onset by only about two months compared to full-term children, while the Norris et al. blind premature subjects—and Kelli and Carlo—fall at the very bottom of the normal range of onset time: eight to twelve months later than the mean for sighted full-term children. These findings begin to suggest that there is an interaction between blindness and prematurity, such that the relatively small effect on language onset associated with prematurity becomes large when it is associated with blindness as well. However, given the state of the evidence—different studies, different measures, etc.—it is not possible to be confident of this interaction or to speculate on its causes. But surely this issue is worth further pursuit.

2. But recall that Kelli and Carlo began to speak later than most sighted children, so the vocabulary data here are from these blind children older—23 (20) and 29 (26) months, respectively—than Nelson's subjects, who ranged from 15 to 24 months.

3. We have discussed overgeneralization at length simply because the charge of "concreteness" has been laid on blind learners by alluding to their alleged narrowness of word usage. But it is important to notice that recent evidence suggests that overgeneralizations and false generalizations are not so common as earlier suspected and thus perhaps cannot carry much weight in developing a theory of lexical concept attainment. Rescorla (1980) collected extensive data on early words and found that

indeed a third of the first 75 vocabulary items were overextended, but that overextension was rare thereafter; moreover, most overgeneralizations were restricted to a categorial close relation (e.g., *ball* for all round things), and some so-called overgeneralizations seemed to be misnomers. For example, the child might say "Dada" when looking at the father's shoe. This kind of usage peaks in frequency (among the uses counted as "overgeneralizations") just before the child starts talking in two-word sentences. As Rescorla notes, the fairest guess is that the child formed no category consisting of the father plus his shoe, but rather was making a first feeble attempt to say something like "Daddy's shoe." Another problem, discussed by Thomson and Chapman (1976), is that many overextensions that occur in early speech fail to occur in comprehension performance by the same individuals, i.e., the overuse of "dog" for many animals may be due more to the small available vocabulary than to a conceptual confusion among the animal species. Finally, Carey has shown in a series of studies (for review, see Carey, 1982) that some apparent overgeneralizations and failures to make distinctions even in comprehension studies may result from the child's inability to concentrate on all implications of a word at once; but when such implications are queried one at a time, the child displays knowledge of them all. In the light of all these interpretive difficulties, along with the practical problems blind children have in pragmatic interpretation of ongoing scenes, it is probably unwise to give apparent spontaneous overgeneralizations too much weight as indicators of the content of their lexical entries.

4. We thank Elissa Newport for making available her data. The MLU measures reported in this section differ slightly for those reported in previous sections. This is because the coding systems of Brown and Newport differed, with Newport crediting the child with inflections using a distributional criterion applied to each separate sample. Since a proper comparison with the sighted data can be made only if the coding is comparable, the data in the prior section were analyzed using Brown's criteria and then reanalyzed for the current analysis using Newport's criteria.

5. We have sketched only a few reflexes of this distinction in language form and use. But it is worth mentioning that the manifestations of the distinction are legion. As further examples, it has been shown that open and closed class emerge separately in language birth (pidgin languages lack closed class resources but gain them under the process of creolization—see Sankoff and Laberge, 1973; Bickerton, 1984). They are lost separately in language death (long-term forgetting of one's native tongue—Dorian, 1978); in this last case, many open-class vocabulary items are forgotten while the closed-class morphology is remembered over periods as long as fifty years of disuse of the language (a fact clearly related to the generalization behind the original naming of these two classes: they are subject to differential forgetting, and thus the class that is not forgotten—the closed class—tends not to change over historical time). Moreover, every known attempt at an explicit parser (machinery that extracts the semantically functioning phrases from arbitrary sen-

tences through syntactic analysis) treats closed-class items distinctively, e.g., as directions for the machinery to move into a new subroutine. Further findings are that the two classes of item are differentially accessible to metalinguistic reflection such as giving judgments of grammaticality or understanding puns (Gleitman and Gleitman, 1979); for closely related reasons, the closed class is especially difficult in such derived language activities as learning to read (Rozin and Gleitman, 1977).

6. Negative imperatives and "polite" imperatives ("Don't eat the daisies" and "Do eat the daisies") have an auxiliary (*do*). Of independent interest is the fact that learning within the open class does not seem to be dependent, like learning of the closed class, on specifiable features of the maternal speech. We have argued elsewhere that this differential sensitivity of the learner to open- and closed-class features of the input data is implicated not only in language learning in the ordinary case but also in properties of self-invented systems of communication among isolated deaf children (Feldman et al., 1978) and in language change (particularly, creolization—see Gleitman and Wanner, 1982; Gleitman et al., 1984). Newport and Supalla (forthcoming) make related claims for their investigations of sign-language users who acquired ASL at different ages.

7. This pattern of learning is particularly striking for two reasons. First, the advantage of yes/no questions for the learner is counterintuitive with respect to what is "simplest" on syntactic and semantic grounds, namely the canonical declarative sentence. Second, what facilitates learning and what gets spoken first by children are different: Children's early utterances of the auxiliaries are within the simple declarative sentences, despite the fact that they seem to be learning about auxiliaries primarily from yes/no questions.

8. There may be further oddities in the blind child's development of what are called conversational skills, i.e., learning how to take turns in speaking with one's conversational partner, etc. However that may be, the work presented here is directed toward the question of how learners solve one formidable problem: discovering the infinite set of sound/meaning pairings that constitute a natural language. For completeness, however, Kelli and Carlo at two years did a lot of rocking of their bodies, saying sentences apparently repeated from earlier conversations without any immediately relevant context, and were late relative to normals in symbolic play, i.e., playing with toys. We believe there is a nondeviant interpretation for these behaviors, though they are usually taken as showing conceptual and emotional deviances (Fraiberg, 1977). For example, the Miss Piggy teapot incident exemplifies the real problem blind two-year-olds have with interpreting objects; no wonder that such icons as dolls and trucks aren't much fun for them at first (though, by 36 months, our subjects seemed to have figured these matters out, and then they did begin to play with toys). As for the "autistic" tendency to utter sentences out of context, we have some preliminary evidence that this is a kind of speech play that functions as the blind equivalent for those missing dolls. Similarly, certain bizarre-looking wiggling and dancing behavior by Kelli (also characteristic of many blind toddlers) seems less

odd when the child is queried. We have some data showing that blind youngsters' pantomiming of motor acts ("Pretend you are eating"), though recognizable in context, looks very strange—the blind child emphasizes in her imitation the parts of the act most salient to the haptic rather than visual perspectives. Caught in some spontaneous motor act, uninterpretable *without* context, inquiry often reveals that a sensible game is going on in the child's head. For instance, we asked Kelli what she was doing when she was performing strange twisting contortions with one hand. In response to "What are you doing?" she said "Having a teaparty. Want some?" The odd physical act, given this context, was retrospectively interpretable as (poorly) mimicking a pouring action by the hand, an act promptly repeated on request, to give us some of the mental tea.

3. The Meaning of Sighted Verbs:
Look as the Blind Child Applies It to Herself

1. It is worth noting that the problem here posed for the investigator is just the problem we are posing for the child learners. Since they too are exposed not to sentence/meaning pairs, but only to utterance/event pairs, different for each learner and for the same learner on different exposures ("learning trials"), how do all of them use these different and indirect clues to reconstruct approximately the same word meanings? In short, how does the extralinguistic context help, since the context is not the meaning? Nonetheless, as the landmark work of Bloom (1970) showed, rich interpretation of the contexts accompanying the young child's language use does seem to provide a reliable data base for making inferences about linguistic intent. And of course, difficult as it is to state *how*, the young child's input of utterance/event pairs in practice does seem to provide a reliable data base for acquiring a grammar. Our aim is to make a contribution to the question of how this gets done in light of the logical difficulties we have reviewed.

2. We have acknowledged that adults have amodal and crossmodal interpretations of the visual verbs: One can use "I hear John isn't doing linguistics these days;" or "I see John isn't doing linguistics these days" to mean the same thing—and in neither case must it be so, for felicity, that one got the information by either seeing or hearing; one may simply have noticed that John is spending all his time surfing. Thus it is of some interest to ask how adults might interpret the various experimental commands in a situation where they are blindfolded. To find out, Mark Schneider (unpublished manuscript) reran all these experiments with undergraduate sighted subjects. These were pilot studies, and in their present form have some procedural warts, but we believe they will stand up in a more formal demonstration.

In the first run of the experiments, ten adults were blindfolded and tested in the sequence presented in the text for Experiments 1, 2, and 5. All of these adults acted just like sighted three-year-olds for about the first twenty questions, after which a few of them switched and began behaving like Kelli, e.g., raising their hands in response to "look up" and sniffing in response to "look with the nose." In a rerun of this work, ten new subjects were warmed up by having them complete simple jigsaw puzzles with their hands after being blindfolded; this was designed to familiarize them with the feeling of being blind and to reveal to them implicitly that the hands could then explore and solve problems previously done mainly by eye. In this new version, the order of questions was varied, because certain of the queries ("look up with your hands") seemed to be more informative than others; perhaps it was the late appearance of these more informative queries that accounted for some of the subjects' late switch in response style. Given these procedural changes, approximately half of the new subjects immediately behaved like Kelli in response to all the questions. The other half behaved as the first ten had: responding like the sighted blindfolded children for some or all of the commands. Though we reiterate that these results must be considered as pilot findings only, they do begin to suggest that even adults are highly biased toward understanding "look" visually. Perhaps "Business looks good" and "I see John isn't doing linguistics" (amodal uses of these words) are metaphorical extensions only, rather than parts of the literal meaning, which may be modal-visual (for this position concerning sighted verbs, see Miller and Johnson-Laird, 1976).

Since these subjects were adults, they did provide one good check on our interpretation of what the three-year-old blindfolded subjects were

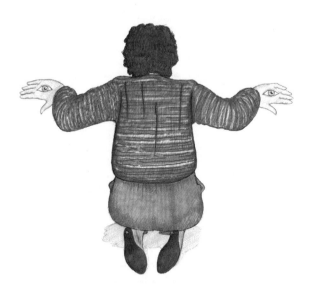

A blindfolded sighted adult's response to "look behind you with your hands." The adult's hands are forward of her body. She behaves as though the hands had grown eyes and that these eyes were looking behind her.

trying to do. The pantomimed behavior of the adults was especially clear, probably because as cooperative subjects they had got through to the idea behind the strange situation and were trying by these panto-mimes to make their comprehension clear to us. For instance, told to "look behind you with your hands," a few subjects held their arms slightly *forward* of the body but out to the sides, turning the palms back-ward, facing behind them as shown in the accompanying Figure. Such a behavior can only be interpreted as the subject making the "visual anal-ogy" which we stated was characteristic of the sighted blindfolded chil-dren too: imagine that an eye has grown in the palm of your hand, and let that new eye look behind you.

4. The Meanings of Sighted Verbs:
Look and *See* as the Blind Child Applies Them to Others

1. Again, the testing was late just because we thought of it late; whether or not Kelli would have performed the same earlier on, i.e., during the three-year old period during which most of the other experi-ments were done, we cannot know.

2. The distinctions here are subtle, and sometimes are honored only in the breech. For example, compare:

(1) I must have looked at that a dozen timés, but I never saw it.

(2) I must have seen that a dozen times, but I never noticed it.

It is obvious that the two sentences differ in the construal of *see: See* in (2) is used as *look* is used in (1). (These examples are from Jackendoff, 1983). As Jackendoff has argued, the looseness of usage is a consequence of the identity of events, ordinarily, in which looking and seeing take place. It is rare to look without seeing or to see without looking, and therefore no difficulty usually arises if the terms are used more or less synonomously. We will return to a fuller discussion of the active/stative distinction in Chapters 5 and 7. For present purposes, it is enough to notice that the distinction is linguistically available in conditions where it is material to the conversation.

3. We thank Susan Scanlon for suggesting this experimental idea to us.

4. Kelli's more openminded approach doubtless is related to her fa-miliarity with conditions of seeing that hold true for sighted people and are untrue of herself. For example, in the natural course of everyday events her mother would sometimes say "I see" when Kelli knew her to be at a distance from some target object or person (but see Chapter 6 for the finding that this knowledge is gained in the presence of only weak and probabilistic extralinguistic evidence). Similarly, a sighted child who lives in an environment with a blind person seems to be approximately as openminded about looking and seeing as Kelli is: Kelli has a sighted sister, Sommer (one year younger than Kelli), whose responses to Kelli were informally observed from the time she was a year old. For the most part, she was sensitive to Kelli's blindness, e.g., putting objects in Kelli's

hands to "show" her or "let her see" them, freely playing with Kelli's toys in front of her, apparently aware that Kelli could not know, etc. When Sommer was 47 months old, we formally tested her behavioral responses to blindness (Landau and Feldman, unpublished manuscript). This experiment mirrored relevant properties of Experiment 2: Sommer was asked to "show" various objects to her blindfolded mother and to "let Mommy see," versus "give" and "let touch." In 12 of 12 trials, regardless of whether the command was about contact (*give/let touch*) or about "seeing" (*show/let see*), she brought the object up close to the blindfolded mother.

6. How Kelli Learned Visual Terms: The Environmental Model

1. The presuppositions of this analysis seem reasonable. They embody the claim that Kelli could (manually, of course) perceive objects. Her early and appropriately used vocabulary of basic object terms (see Table 2.1) provide a *prima facie* case for this assumption. Also they embody the claim that she could determine the spatial-locational properties of objects relative to her own body. The bases for this claim are her early and appropriate use of locative prepositions such as *up*, which appear among her earliest words (see again Table 2.1) and her correct responses to queries about them (as shown in Chapter 3 and 4). Further evidence for her spatial knowledge early in development was provided by observation of her competence in navigating her home environment and during explicit study of her spatial inferences (Landau et al., 1981, 1984).

2. The case of *You look funny* is quite complex. Though the sentence starts out *You look . . .* it is not the case that the referent of the subject NP (in this case, Kelli) is asserted to be looking at all. Rather, notionally *you* (Kelli) is the object being inspected, even though it is the subject NP in the sentence. It is the speaker (in this case, the mother) who is looking, and the predicate is something like 'appear funny by my (the mother's) visual inspection.' The semantics and syntax of such uses of *look* are taken up in detail in Chapter 7. Here we make the plausible assumption that a toddler learning *look* is no party to these complexities in interpreting this usage.

3. Some objections can be raised to this analysis, for perhaps it grants too much inferential capacity to the learner. The question is whether we have a right to assume that Kelli is in a position to determine a target object of looking (e.g., the boot) when it is not explicitly mentioned in the sentence that contains the word *look*. Since we did not know, we performed a second analysis requiring that the target object be present (in the child's hand or near it) and *also* that it be mentioned in the sentence containing the verb. As it turned out, the results of this analysis were not interestingly different from the one presented in the text. But for completeness the results of this additional analysis appear here:

Spatial versus Linguistic Coding of Verbs[a]

Verb	Hand + Near		Far		No object	
	+Ling. object	−Ling. object	+Ling. object	−Ling. object	+Ling. object	−Ling. object
Perceptual verbs						
Look	.50	.22	.00	.08	.14	.06
See	.33	.06	.44	.11	.00	.06
Nonperceptual verbs						
Come	.00	.05	.00	.32	.00	.63
Get	.45	.05	.20	.05	.00	.25
Give	.97	.00	.03	.00	.00	.00
Go	.00	.52	.10	.14	.00	.24
Have	.53	.00	.33	.14	.00	.00
Hold	1.00	.00	.00	.00	.00	.00
Play	.50	.20	.00	.00	.30	.00
Put	.97	.00	.00	.00	.03	.00
Say	.43	.00	.07	.00	.50	.00

a. Spatial coding categories are the same as those used in previous tables (see Table 6.2 and text for discussion). Linguistic coding categories include (a) sentences where a NP is mentioned (+Ling. object), as in "See Barbara's boot?"; and (b) sentences where a NP is not mentioned (−Ling. object), as in "See?," though an object might be nearby and it might have been easy to infer that action on that object was intended.

The numbers in this table are slightly different from those in Table 6.2, as a consequence of rounding over six rather than three categories here.

4. More precisely, this is true of only one of two readings of *get*. There is a sense of *get*, the one we are here concerned with, that is quite passive and means something like *receive*. When someone gives you something, willy-nilly you receive it in this sense. Getting the Nobel Prize is a case of this sort. You do not apply for the prize but simply receive it on the basis of decisions made by others. (The IRS makes the same distinction between the two readings of *get* and thus, since one doesn't apply, holds that Nobel Prize money is nontaxable.) But sometimes *get* is used more actively. Consider *getting a Ph.D.* You get it from the university authorities in the same sense that you get the Nobel Prize from the appropriate Swedish authorities. But there is another sense of *getting a Ph.D.*: You perform certain voluntary acts such as writing a thesis. A sentence like *John got a Ph.D* thus invites at least slightly different inferences when said by the university registrar and when said by the candidate's proud mother.

5. It is important to realize that the mother's speech to Kelli consists primarily of commands and requests directed to her, as we showed in Chapter 2. This is why this analysis can work: When the mother says "Give the boot. . .", the boot is near Kelli. If instead the corpus were replete with declarative comments such as "Your father gave a dollar to the United Way," the analysis for the position of target objects would have

failed even more generally. But even this does not suggest that the near/far analysis would have been irrelevant to Kelli's learning. Her job in this new situation would be to select only verb uses in which she herself was mentioned explicitly in the sentence (or, in the imperative, implied), or at least to select as relevant to learning only those events for which she could determine the relative positions of the objects and persons who figured in the heard sentence.

6. It is worth noting that other proposals for the discovery of sentence meaning and verb meaning in particular similarly presuppose such a global parse of simple sentences. As one example, see Braine and Hardy's "case grammar" proposal (1982). In their model, the learner makes conjectures about predicate-argument structure, based on a presupposed ability to determine the number and positions of NPs, relative to the verb, in the sentence. The present proposal makes the weaker assumption that the child can determine the number and positions of NPs, but does not know how their placement in the string maps onto the verb arguments.

7. In further detail, the ordered list of categories that can follow a particular verb, and that represent the arguments of the verb, is what we mean by the verb's subcategorization frame. It is necessary for a grammar to list these frames as part of the lexical entry for a verb just because they cannot be wholly accounted for in any general way, for example, as simple derivatives of a semantic scheme that describes predicate-argument structure. This can be seen from the examples just given: The idea of vanishing a rabbit (causing a rabbit to vanish) is not bizarre, at least for magicians. And for many verbs of English (though not *vanish*), causative ideas are expressed with simple transitive verbs, as in *to sink a ship, melt a candle*. Disallowing this possibility for *vanish* is evidently an arbitrary structural restriction for this verb. Thus, though we shall argue at length in Chapter 7 that there are stable relations between the subcategorization frames and the logic of verb meanings (that syntactic properties of sentences carry significant semantic information), there may be an arbitrary component as well (see Grimshaw, 1983, for discussion). If so, the subcategorization frames must be stored as lexical (item-specific) information. Verbs usually accept more than one such frame, e.g., *give* accepts both NP PP (*I gave a book to John*) and NP NP (*I gave John a book*). In a descriptive scheme that, to account for the meaning relations between two frames that apply to a single verb, relates the two frames in the lexical entry (a scheme we will adopt in Chapter 7), the NPs are subscripted so as to keep track of which is which. For example, for *give* we might render the subcategorization frames as ——— (NP_1) (P NP_2) and ——— (NP_2) (NP_1), where the parentheses stand for phrase boundaries (see Bresnan, 1978). These paired entries can render information about sentential relations that in early versions of generative grammar (Chomsky, 1965) were described by transformations. We assume further that each preposition represents a distinct syntactic category, much like the postpositional case markings of many other languages, such as Latin; for evidence that children make these crucial distinctions among the

prepositions very early in the learning process, see Table 2.1, which shows locative prepositions among the earliest 50 words in Kelli and Carlo's vocabularies. Thus, for example, the frame underlying *John gave a book to Mary* includes the information that the P in the phrase *to Mary* is *to*.

8. The presupposition of the present analysis, of course, is that the child learner performs equivalent codings of heard utterances. Therefore the learner must confront the same problems that we just suggested were faced by the coders of these data. For example, the learner will hear many PPs that are really parts of NPs ("the brother *of John*") or optional modifiers of the sentence as a whole ("I saw my uncle *on Monday*"). In short, many nominal and prepositional phrases that look for all the world like arguments of the verb are not. How is the learner to realize this? As we will discuss more fully in Chapter 7, clues come from the prosody of the utterance (see, e.g., Cooper and Paccia-Cooper, 1980, for evidence that there are prosodic cues in the speech wave that disambiguate these prepositional phrases, providing a basis on which they can be assigned distinctive bracketing—and hence labelling—in the parse of the heard sentence; and Read and Schreiber, 1982, for evidence that children use these prosodic cues to structure). Of course life would be much harder for a child who had to learn English by reading rather than listening.

9. The counterexample, as shown in the table, is a causative use of *have*. It is also true, as the table shows, that only *see* occurs with *come* as an auxiliary ("Come see what I have"), but this is surely just a glitch in the utterance sample. Unlike the other restrictions of format being discussed, this is not a syntactic property true of the language at large: It is natural to say "Come get the horse," and so on.

10. See note 3 to Chapter 7 for a discussion of reciprocal verbs such as *play, collide,* and *argue.*

7. Syntactic and Ostensive Supports for Verb Learning

1. We thank Rochel Gelman for reminding us of the interesting findings from Lenneberg and for suggesting the noncoincidental relationship between rapid lexical concept attainment and the appearance of syntactically organized speech.

2. Maratsos (1982) and Levy (1983a), discussing the German and Hebrew (nonnatural) gender systems, point out that very young children can extract form-class distinctions that are semantically incoherent. Nonetheless, we believe that the semantic bootstrapping hypothesis does much of the required work of getting the child into the language system.

3. The issues here are more complex than we have acknowledged so far. We now attempt a more detailed general analysis of evidently "symmetrical" and "asymmetrical" predicates, asking how these readings are marked in the surface structures of English (for an early statement of these ideas, see Gleitman, 1965; for a quite different account of the same verb domain, see McCawley, 1970). We will also discuss some of the se-

mantic properties that determine the placement of nominal arguments under the asymmetric readings. As is standard in linguistic discussion, we consider the fact that certain of these predicates are expressed adjectively (e.g., *is similar to* and *is equal to*) while others are expressed as verbs (e.g., *resembles* and *equals*) a surface property of rather minor interest; therefore we ignore this distinction in the following discussion.

Does the asymmetry of a predicate determine the order of NPs in surface structure? In the text, we discussed the case of *similar*, which is interpreted symmetrically in certain syntactic configurations but not in others. To repeat, (1) and (2) below are interpreted asymmetrically while (3)–(5) are interpreted symmetrically (Tversky, 1977).

(1) North Korea is similar to China.
(2) China is similar to North Korea.
(3) China and North Korea are similar to each other.
(4) China and North Korea are similar.
(5) North Korea and China are similar.

Tversky extended this analysis to the predicate *differ* as well. Tversky's interest in the construal of these predicates centrally has to do with the topic of human categorization performance, for which it is crucial to understand the sense or senses in which humans take individual items to be alike enough to group them together for some or all purposes. His plausible interpretation of the difference between sentences (1) and (2) had to do with the relative prototypicality of, e.g., China and North Korea, under some categorization which the listener could induce from the pair itself (in this case, "countries," as Tversky showed in further experiments). Roughly, *similar* in (1) and (2) seems to be interpreted as a case of comparing some exemplar (North Korea) against a standard or prototypical exemplar (China); since China is the likely standard, sentence (2) seems less natural and leads to judgments of a lesser degree of similarity. For this verb, then, evidently the standard appears as the postverbal NP. For the cases of (3)–(5), neither NP is set up as the standard, i.e., the similarity relation is symmetrical.

Here our purposes are to ask about the generality of the judgmental phenomena investigated by Tversky (though we present only examples, no experimental data), and to relate them to the linguistic system that encodes them in English.

In our view, the problem with *similar* is not altogether resolved by Tversky's claim that this is (surprisingly) an asymmetric verb for which a symmetrical reading (as in 3) is just a special case. Consider the following dramatic instances from Talmy (1983):

(6) The bicycle is near the garage.
(7) ?The garage is near the bicycle.
(8) ?The bicycle and the garage are near each other.

It doesn't seem that *near* has any asymmetric reading. The bicycle cannot be nearer to the garage than the garage is to the bicycle. Yet sentence (7) and particularly (8) are problematical, and doubtless subjects could be induced to judge them of different "naturalness." In this case, the natural order does not seem to reside in the relative prototypicality or standardness of garages versus bicycles or people versus trees. Rather it seems clear that it is the relative size and mobility of the objects and the focus of a geometrical layout that determine the natural order of the two NPs. Moreover the directionality cannot be cancelled by use of the *each other* construction, which remains odd no matter the attempted construal (see Talmy for this example and a full discussion). As these samples begin to show, there are a variety of bases for the ordering of NPs relative to the predicate. Prototypicality may be the one for *similar*, but size and mobility (*tie, near*) and cause (e.g., *kiss, introduce, hit*) are among the many others. Thus a particular argument order may be mandated in the syntax of the language independent of the symmetry of the predicate but dependent instead on other aspects of the relation between the arguments (stability, mobility, cause, etc.; again see Talmy for discussion). As this claim implies, it is possible that there is a difference in naturalness of NP ordering even for the most prototypical of all symmetrical predicates; compare:

(9) The least of the citizens of the nation is equal to the President of the United States.

(10) ?The President of the United States is equal to the least of the citizens of the nation.

Encoding symmetrical and asymmetrical interpretations of a predicate syntactically. Three kinds of predicate must be considered to understand the properties of *similar*. One is the large set that, in virtue of its logic, allows no symmetrical reading in any frame. For example, in

(11) John hit Mary
(12) Mary hit John

the reading must be asymmetric; (11) doesn't entail (12), nor does the one sentence pragmatically invite an inference to the other, even if Mary is known to be a violent and vengeful type. As we shall describe, the inherent asymmetry of the predicate *hit* predicts that there is no further form

(13) *John and Mary hit

with the symmetrical logical interpretation

(14) John hit Mary and Mary hit John.

In contrast, there is a very large number of predicates like *similar*, including such common cases as *kiss, argue, meet, fight, play, struggle, resemble,* and *collide*. These are asymmetrical in such formats as

(15) John kissed Mary
(16) The bus collided with the car

but symmetrical in such formats as

(17) John and Mary kissed
(18) The car and the bus collided.

For example, it would be natural to say (16) if the front of the bus hit the side of the car (i.e., if the bus caused the collision), but unnatural to say

(19) The car collided with the bus

under these circumstances.

As for (18), it is probably most naturally reserved to head-on collisions, in which case

(20) The bus and the car collided

is a natural alternative sentence. Notice, then, that though *hit* and *collide* are very close in meaning, they differ in the respect that the latter and not the former has intransitive forms—(13) is anomalous while (18) is not— and moreover intransitive uses of *collide* require a plural or conjoined subject (e.g., **The bus collided* is as odd as **John hit*).

It should be noted that the subcategorization of a verb's subject NP (for *collide*, the requirement of a plural NP) as a function of its object (for *collide*, the plural subject is required only if there is no direct object) is rare: To our knowledge, only the kind of predicates we are now discussing have this surface property. We shall argue that this is no exception to the general rule that verbs subcategorize for objects independent of subjects, for (17) and (18) will not in our scheme be listed among the subcategorization frames for these verbs.

Summarizing the direction we will take at this point, probably we do not want, for *collide* or *kiss* any more than for *similar*, to adjudicate the question of symmetry of interpretation by reference to the predicate in isolation. Rather, symmetry for each of hundreds of English verbs is a logical property that can be read off some, but not all, the surface formats in which such verbs appear. If this is true, merely assigning symmetry or nonsymmetry as a semantic value to the particular predicate *similar* misses a number of significant generalizations: First, we would want our theory to handle not only this particular verb, but the many scores of verbs, e.g., *kiss, argue,* and *collide*, which behave just like *similar* in the relevant regards. Second, the assignment of the semantic value 'asymmetry' fails taken alone to account for the symmetrical readings of (3) and (4) as opposed to the asymmetrical reading of (1) and (2). Third, this assignment of a semantic value taken alone suggests that *similar* is no different in this regard from *hit* by ignoring the fact that *similar* has logical relations to such verbs as *equate* and *match* while *hit* does not. Fourth, it fails to account for why the verbs we are considering, unlike the mass of English predicates, require plural or conjoined subjects only when they are used intransitively (i.e., **The woman met* is odd, but *The women met* is unexceptional).

Given all these descriptive failures, we propose a different analysis, one that if correct will subsume all these verbs and predict their varying construals in sentences that differ in format.

For all transitive "reversible" verbs (those that can take the same kinds of items as their subjects and objects, cf. Slobin, 1966), one can construct sentences with *each other* that notionally are a special kind of conjunction, termed a reciprocal conjunction. For example,

(21) John and Mary kissed each other
(22) John and Mary hit each other

are ways of saying

(23) John kissed Mary and Mary kissed John
(24) John hit Mary and Mary hit John.

Suppose we claim that for certain verbs it is possible to omit the phrase containing *each other*, e.g., (21) and (23) can also be rendered as (17). In contrast, for a much larger set of verbs the omission of *each other* is uniformly disallowed, i.e., (13) is not shorthand for (22) or (24). If this analysis is accepted, we can state the lexical entries for the verbs under discussion and account for their apparently varying construals. They are entered into the lexicon with a single subcategorization frame, e.g., for *hit* and *kiss* this will be

(25) NP_1 V NP_2

However, for *kiss* (and *similar*) but not *hit*, a semantic feature RECIP is entered as well. As we shall show, this feature comes into play in deriving the logical form of certain sentences containing *kiss* and *similar*, but not in all sentences containing these words.

There may be a third class of predicates that have symmetrical readings only (e.g., *equal, match, identical*), though examples (9) and (10) may suggest that this class is empty. Insofar as the idea that there are some uniformly symmetrical verbs is correct, the choice of surface frame has no effect on the construal or on the inferences it invites:

(26) This rug matches this sofa.
(27) This sofa matches this rug.
(28) This sofa and this rug match each other.
(29) This sofa and this rug match.

all probably have the same meaning and invite the same inferences, i.e., all these sentences strictly entail one another. To model this property, we enter a pair of subcategorization frames, namely those underlying (26) and (27) for such verbs. In addition, the specification RECIP appears in their lexical entries.

Notice that nothing has so far been said about frames underlying sentences (3)–(5) and such other examples as (17), (20), (28), and (29). We suggest that none of these frames is specified for any verb in the lexicon. Rather, we propose that these structures arise from a rule of construal (or a syntactic rule, depending on the grammar chosen) that interprets reciprocal conjunctions for every verb that can choose the same kind of entity for two of its NP argument positions. This is a property of English that is constructive just like the rules that derive conjunctions with *and, or,* and *but*, and it is about as broad in applicability; it is a required component of the description of English independent of the need to describe symmetrical verbs. The rule refers to the classification of nominal types just as do all rules of conjunction (e.g., *I love Robert and fishing* and *Robert and fishing are similar to each other* are odd on related grounds, though occasionally nominals of quite different types are marginally acceptable in such constructions, e.g., while *Robert and Nora disagree with each other* is the more natural kind of usage, *Robert and hard liquor disagree with each other* is perhaps possible).

This much information in hand, we can now describe how reciprocal conjunction will run given the trifurcation of the predicates earlier described: predicates that are always symmetrical (*equate, match, identical,* which list a pair of entailment frames and the specification RECIP), those that are asymmetrical (*similar, kiss, collide,* and list a single frame plus the specification RECIP), and those that are asymmetrical (*hit, stop, eat,* and list a single frame without the specification RECIP): Simply, the specification RECIP optionally triggers (or interprets, again depending on the machinery adopted) deletion of the node dominating *each other* in reciprocal conjunctions (and by the general linguistic convention of pruning, everything under the deleted node automatically deletes as well). For example,

(30) John and Mary argue with each other

is optionally rendered as

(31) John and Mary argue w̶i̶t̶h̶ ̶e̶a̶c̶h̶ ̶o̶t̶h̶e̶r̶

The result is the tree shown below.

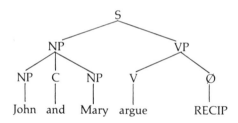

How can this result in a nondirectional reading at the level of logical form? The first part of the answer is that (31) now has the form of a conjunction with *and*. The semantic value of *and* is always nondirectional, no matter the lexical or syntactic rule through which it is inserted into sentential structures, and hence (31) receives a coordinate interpretation (recall that semantic interpretation in recent grammars is on the surface or S-structures, not on the underlying forms).

But this is not quite enough. All we so far know is that *and* implies a coordinate relation between *John* and *Mary* in (30) and (31). But is that coordination reciprocal? Notice that (31), unlike (30), is ambiguous: It could mean that John and Mary both argue (with some unspecified other) or that they argue with each other. For verbs like *similar* and *meet,* which are entered as pure transitives in the mental dictionary, the intransitive forms could have arisen from reciprocal conjunction only (hence their intransitive plural or conjoined forms are unambiguous, and their intransitive singulars are ungrammatical); but for verbs like *argue* (which can be used both transitively and intransitively), conjoined *and* plural intransitives are ambiguous as between ordinary and reciprocal conjunction, and their singular intransitives are grammatical. Of course, at the level of S-structure, as the tree shows, the difference in interpretation is exhibited; nonetheless, there is an ambiguity for the listener if the verb chosen is *argue*, but not if it is *meet* (a pure transitive) or *hit* (which is not marked for RECIP) or *square*, as in *The mathematician squared the circle* (which specifies different kinds of entities for its subject [animate] and its object [inanimate] and therefore is blocked from reciprocal conjunction).

In sum, we have posited that English has a rule of reciprocal conjunction which can apply to all so-called reversible predicates: those that can take the same kind of entity as their subjects and objects. Notice that a predicate may be notionally symmetrical (e.g., *near*) and still not reversible in this sense: As we described earlier, *near* requires a relatively large and immobile entity in the first NP position and a more mobile one in the second NP position; this distinction of entity type for subject and object position predicts the absence of a reciprocal conjunction, i.e., the oddity of (8). Further, we postulated a semantic property (RECIP) that triggers pruning of the node dominating *each other* in reciprocal conjunctions. This machinery can model the fact that in some structures, namely the pruned *each other* constructions, pure transitive verbs have only symmetrical construals. Subsidiary supports for this argument are that it predicts the fact that surface forms for predicates such as *match* and *meet* can occur intransitively (without an NP as direct object) just in case their subjects are plural or conjoined. We proposed that only the true symmetrical verbs (if these exist) will accept the symmetrical reading at the level of logical form outside reciprocal conjunctions; this would be modelled by paired subcategorization frames in the lexical entry for *equal* or *match*. Thus the verbs we have been discussing are prime cases where properties of surface form transparently render the logical form. They show as well a general case in which all the surface syntactic facts, not a subcategorization frame taken in isolation, can be informative to a learner in extracting that logic. In contrast, it is difficult to say anything coherent or general about this class of predicates without attention to all their surface frames.

4. "Freely" is really too strong a term here: There are important restrictions on which locative prepositions can occur with which motion verbs, as Gruber has shown. We shall return to these distinctions later, where we show the differences between *look* and *see*. An important detail, described in note 3, is the construction *play with X*. *With* is here a relational particle, and the predicate *play* participates in the reciprocal structure described in the note.

5. Notice that the special sports usage, *look the ball into one's hands*, does not mean 'cause the ball to go into the hands by looking.' This is an impossible idea, unless you believe in psychokinesis. Rather, it means 'look at the ball all the way until it reaches your hands' (probably also impossible, given limitations on visual tracking performances, but more or less possible for wide receivers who are better than others at catching the ball that hits their hands).

6. Recall that there was a single other case of a common verb in the corpus taking a sentential complement (see Table 6.3). This is the utterance "Let's have Miss Barbara over to babysit," in which *have* appears as a causative (and sensibly enough, for one can cause events to occur just as one can perceive events to occur). This shows, as we shall discuss later, that a single subcategorization frame is not informative enough for selecting a particular lexical interpretation; the appearance of *see* with a sentential complement is not sufficient to assign it a perceptual rather than causative interpretation, but only begins to narrow down the field (e.g., it cannot simply be a verb of physical motion). We have already mentioned supportive further information in the data base which is available for accomplishing these further refinements: *Have,* but not *see,* has been excluded from the set of motion verbs on the basis of the restriction in locative prepositional phrases (the absence of *Have it on the table,* etc.). Similarly, the apparatus already mentioned is sufficient for distinguishing between *see* and many other mental verbs such as *think, suspect, want, realize,* and *hope.* Again, the grounds are that these do not have the syntactic characteristics of motion verbs, such as free use with locative prepositions and adverbs. It is a set of cross-cutting syntactic cues that is doing the work.

7. A complication with the verb *get* at first glance seems to defeat the generalization just described, but ends by strengthening it. Notice that in Table 6.3 there were a number of uses of *get* in subcategorization frames no different from those just described for *come* and *look.* These include usages such as *Get up.* But as the subcategorization frames for these verbs become more alike, so do their meanings. *Get up* is notionally not far from *Go up.* In further detail, we have concentrated some attention on the motion verbs *come* and *go,* which express the inalienable movements of their subjects. There are of course semantic relatives of these verbs which (like *give*) also express the alienable agent: *bring* (*John brings Mary* means 'John is the agent who effects Mary's coming') and *take* (*John takes Mary* means 'John is the agent who effects Mary's going'). *Get* is a case for which the causative and the noncausative are expressed by a single lexical form (e.g., *John got Mary up, Mary got up*), rather than by a pair (such as *bring/come* and *take/go*). There are many parallel instances in English (e.g., *John sank the ship, The ship sank*). Notice, in addition, that even the notion of movement in *see* can appear in structures, perhaps awkward but certainly intelligible, in which the gaze is treated as an alienable object, for example by using Gruber's own locution, *move the gaze toward.* One can say "John moved his gaze toward the door" or "John held his gaze steady." In these cases, John is treated as the agent who effects the movement, the gaze is now (metaphorically) an alienable object that is moved, and it is moved toward the door. But in these structures, it is the case that there is an extra NP (*his gaze*) in the sentences, the one that represents the alienable object.

8. As we have stated earlier, the present progressive is much more natural with active verbs (*I am looking at the moon*) than with stative verbs (*I am seeing the moon*), but the prohibition against progressives with sta-

tives is not honored very exactly either by Kelli or by her mother. This property is known to be learned late by children (see Gleitman, Gleitman, and Shipley, 1972, for some evidence), but it is mildly surprising that her mother does sometimes say to Kelli "Are you seeing that?" *Look* does of course occur in the progressive both in the maternal and child corpus (e.g., the mother says "Keep looking").

9. Some verbs seem at first glance to be synonymous, and yet they differ in their surface forms. We will try to show that at least sometimes the appearance of synonymy is at least in part illusory, that the difference in subcategorization frames can be identified with (and, indeed, describes) a subtle distinction in the construals of semantically related verbs.

The verbs we consider are *replace* and *substitute*, mentioned by Grimshaw (1983) as prime examples of semantic arbitrariness in the assignment of subcategorization frames. Surely Grimshaw is correct in asserting that these two verbs are very similar in meaning: Both encode, much in the same way, events in which some agent effects the removal of some entity and the insertion of another in its place. Yet though they share three-argument structure formats, as would be predicted from this sense, they differ in the preposition each takes in the oblique argument position and in the placement of the two nonagentive arguments. For example:

(1) John substitutes a mouse for a rat.
(2) John replaces a rat with a mouse.

One can omit one of the oblique arguments of *replace*.

(3) John replaces a rat. (an entailment of 2)

The omission of an oblique argument of *substitute* sounds rather more awkward, and in any case it is a different argument that is omitted:

(4) ?John substitutes a mouse. (an entailment of 1)
(5) *John substitutes a rat. (as an entailment of 1)

The agent can be omitted for each of these verbs, maintaining entailment relations, but the subcategorization frames again look different:

(6) A mouse substitutes for a rat. (an entailment of 1)
(7) A mouse replaces a rat. (an entailment of 2)

A further effect of these patterns is that sentences such as (3) and (7) are ambiguous as to whether the first argument (leftmost NP) is agent or not. It could be that (7) means that the mouse replaces the rat with something else (say, an aardvark) in the sense of (3) or that the mouse takes the place previously held by the mouse—the intended sense of (7) in our example.

Clearly, then, the subcategorization frames for these two verbs differ. Yet this distinction does not seem to be arbitrary. Rather, it is associated with a subtle distinction between their construals: The focus of *replace* is on the entity removed, while the focus of *substitute* is on the entity that is inserted, as is shown both by which of the two oblique arguments may be omitted when the agent appears in the surface structure (compare 3 and 4, each of which omits the nonfocussed argument position), and also by the natural questions and answers associated with sentences in which they appear. Consider again the (same) event associated with sentences (1) and (2). We can ask: "What did you replace?" and the natural answer can only be "a rat," but if we ask "What did you substitute?" the answer must be "a mouse." Thus presence of the pair *replace/substitute* in English is thus perhaps not an accidental case of synonymy, but rather a lexical distinction that allows the emphasis or perspective taken on the same event to be placed in different ways—in this case, either on the entity that goes away or on the one that is inserted in its place.

We have proposed that there is a semantic correlate to the subcategorization distinctions between these two verbs. Still, there are at least two reasons to question whether speaker-listeners actually represent the subcategorization relations between them systematically. The first has to do with the complexity of the construal rules that would be necessary (e.g., the second argument of *substitute* maps onto the third argument of *replace*, notionally). The second has to do with the breadth of applicability of this postulated lexical rule. Often—or so we have argued—such rules apply very broadly across the verb lexicon, but for the *substitute/replace* relation, the applicability is quite narrow, extending to such pairs as *rob/steal* (one robs John of money and steals money from John) and *inform/announce* (one informs John of the decision and announces the decision to John), but perhaps not much further. (We thank L. Naigles and R. Ostrin for suggesting these further cases.) It is quite possible that complex construal rules whose applicability is restricted to a narrow subclass of the verbs might be ignored by learners, who would instead simply store the information about these subcategorization frames as a semantically arbitrary choice (just as Grimshaw supposes). Of course our proposals about *learning* verbs depend crucially on there being rules of construal that apply broadly across the set of verbs.

10. An important detail is that not all verb frames need be listed separately in the verb entry: Some of them can be generated by lexical redundancy rules much as discussed by Bresnan (1978). For example, within stateable limits, transitive verbs appear in passive constructions, so the passive forms need not be listed for each verb at its individual entry. Rather, the redundancy rules operate on all lexical entries that meet their categorial specifications, often a very wide range of items.

11. See Gleitman and Gleitman, 1970, for evidence that speakers do differ significantly in their constructive lexical representations, though probably not in their syntactic representations. For example, some speakers think that the idea 'dog who brings the mail' should be expressed as "mail-dog" but others think "dog mail-man." That is, *mailman* is a simple word for some speakers but has substructure for others.

12. This contrasts with compositional approaches to the semantics of nouns (for views pro and con, see Katz, 1972, and Fodor, 1981). Evidence for the decomposition of nouns in sentence comprehension or perception has certainly been hard to come by (J. D. Fodor, J. A. Fodor, and

Garrett, 1975; Fodor, Garrett, Walker, and Parkes, 1980). However, the sense of decomposability for predicates we have tried to defend is different. We have taken the orthodox view that the semantics of the predicate is in terms of a predicate-argument logic, and the (only slightly less orthodox) view that this logic is marked in the surface structures of sentences. This marking is complex and, to be sure, there may be an arbitrary component, as we shall discuss further. Still, the stable correlations between the subcategorization choices of verbs and components of the meanings they convey support the reality of these components, in our view. We agree with Fodor and his colleagues that, in contrast, the posited sublexical "features" or "elements" of nouns have yet to be demonstrated. Not only is there a lack of supportive evidence in studies of learning and sentence processing; the posited features for nouns are not indicated with any generality in the forms of sentences. To be sure, verbs differentially select for semantic properties of their noun phrases, and attempts have been made to reconstruct a featural description of the nouns from such evidence (Katz and Fodor, 1963). But, as Fodor (1983) later argued, this effort has not been very successful.

13. Though we are accepting Gruber's analysis in this discussion, there may be a semantic generalization—rather than an arbitrary subcategorization factor—behind the behavior of *see* in this regard. For the active verb of audition, *listen*, there is also a preposition (*to*), and for the stative, *hear*, there is not; for an active verb of olfaction, *sniff*, there is a preposition (*at*), while for *smell* there is not. So this may be a systematic fact about the encoding of perceptual verbs in English (Fillmore, 1968). We cannot defend such a view in any detail, however. For example, if this is a semantically motivated subcategorization choice, it should be expected that active *touch* would take a preposition, perhaps *touch on* or *touch to*, but it does not. Owing to this apparent inconsistency, we must assume that Gruber is correct in his description of *see*, as we have reported it in the text. But perhaps the last word has not been said on this matter.

14. There is a historical reason for this oddity, to be sure, so it is the kind of exception that at least bears on the rule. The in (*en-*) and out (*ex-*) components of *enter* and *exit* were once morphologically exhibited in the surface form. But today it would be surprising if English speakers recognized these morphological variants of the usual prepositional markers (see again note 11). So unless the learner is an etymologist, these cases should put him in something of a pickle.

15. We do not mean to overstate the coherence of these forms mothers use. Johansson (unpublished manuscript) has evidence that the range of maternal descriptions for, e.g., the part-whole distinction, is greater in natural speech than in the picture-naming task used by the investigators we have cited. Further, the use of the genitive pronominal (*his*) does not distinguish between alienable and inalienable possession, i.e., body parts of snakes but also hats that snakes are wearing are often spoken of in the same way: "Here is a snake; these are his eyes" and "Here is a snake; this is his hat." Thus though the maternal speech forms are doubtless infor-

mative, it is also doubtless that it takes a little tact and sophistication to avoid false inductions they may make available.

16. Having raised these alternatives to our own analysis, it is important to note that maybe they are not so plausible. First, the idea is not so attractive, considering known constraints on babies' ability to store and manipulate huge data stores, that the child keeps track of the whole list of nouns that occurs with each verb, a requirement if the "holdable" versus "look-at-able" analysis is to work (in contrast to the syntactic frame analysis, which involves depositing a small number of abstract specifications for a verb, rather than holding any of its particular uses—specific sentences—in memory). Moreover, this distinction does not seem promising for the blind child in particular. For the sighted, there are myriad things one might be told to look at but never told to hold (mountains, birds, the sky). For the blind child, these distinctions largely disappear.

8. A Blind Child's Understanding of Color Terms

1. In a period succeeding the time when Experiment 8.3 was conducted when Kelli was four years old, she did receive a new set of objects that would have been subject to this blocking of an induction through an organized set of counterexamples. Odd as this may seem, blind children including Kelli are often given braille-coded crayons; she even learned to scrawl on paper with them! Here color is coded in terms of dot patterns, rather than in terms of sizes, as of the rings. For the crayons, Kelli was in a position to notice that same-sized objects can receive different color labels. However, we know of no such setting, present in the period when Kelli was offered the stacking rings, that could have played this role and thus explained her behavior in Experiment 8.3. It is an open question, then, whether there might nevertheless have been useful counterexamples during the three-year-old period, organized enough for Kelli to consider in learning a real-world mapping of color terms.

2. Locke's view was more subtle than we have acknowledged, and indeed in some ways is quite consistent with the claim we are making. Locke certainly held the impeccable view that the color qualia are given to the visual sense alone, and that these qualia cannot be ascertained through any other sense. In this respect, a blind man cannot know color. (In fact, Locke specifically rejects the claim of a blind acquaintance of his that this person could know of color by certain analogies: The blind person says that, after all, the meaning *red* is like the sound of a trumpet, and Locke finds this worse than uncompelling—rather, a demonstration of the fact that the blind know nothing at all about color.) We have argued in this chapter that the blind learner knows something about the structure of the category *color* all the same (e.g., that it is related to such domains as *length* in applying only to concrete objects, and is internally organized by the warm/cool distinction). In one passage, Locke forcefully argues that after all knowledge of the structure of a domain may be more important than identification of the qualia: *"Though one Man's Idea of Blue should be different from another's.* Neither would it carry any imputa-

tion of falsehood to our simple ideas, if by the different structure of our organs it was so ordered that *the same object should produce in several men's minds different ideas* at the same time; v.g., if the idea that a violet produced in one man's mind by his eyes were the same that a marigold produced in another man's and *vice versa*. For, since this could never be known, because one man's mind could not pass into another man's body, to perceive what appearances were produced by those organs, neither the ideas hereby, nor the names, would be at all confounded, or any falsehood be in either. For all things, that had the texture of a violet producing constantly the idea which he called blue, and those which had the texture of a marigold producing constantly that which he as constantly called yellow, whatever these appearances were in his mind, he would be able as regularly to distinguish things for his use by those appearances, and understand and signify those distinctions marked by the names 'blue' and 'yellow', as if the appearances or ideas in his mind received from those two flowers were exactly the same with the ideas in other men's minds" (Book 2.XXXII.15).

9. Speculations on the Concept 'Natural Concept'

1. Locke acknowledged that some, though not all, ideas (concepts) could be acquired equivalently from the evidence of more than one sense, as our previous citation concerning the acquisition of *statue* by a blind man suggests. But Berkeley (1709) seems to have taken a stricter view of this matter: "The extension, figures, and motions perceived by sight are specifically distinct from the ideas of touch, called by the same names, nor is there any such thing as one idea, or kind of idea, common to both senses" (sec. 127).

2. One could of course seek to defend the idea that despite the similarities in items learned, course of the learning, and use of the learned items in conversation, the underpinnings of the lexical concepts are somehow systematically different for the blind and sighted learners. However, in the language-learning literature it is usually granted that a learner has acquired a word, say *duck*, insofar as he utters that word in response to ducks, and selects ducks in response to that word. The same evidence exists for Carlo and Kelli. So whatever the status of such evidence, it is no less secure for the one population than for the other. At any rate, there is no real way to evaluate the claim that blind children have different lexical concepts, despite their apposite use of words, in the absence of some lexical theory that could describe just how this could happen and of what the blind person's "novel" vocabulary items might consist, in contrast to our own.

3. Such ideas die hard. Consider again the claims from Werth (1983) that we mention in our preface. Werth argues, without evidence, that "the sad fact is that the language of Kelli and children like her is *inevitably* deficient" because "for blind people there is an area of experience which can never be detailed at first hand." Though he acknowledges that

much—even most—human language is abstract (nonperceptual) anyway and hence poses analogous problems to any learner, he asserts with puzzling confidence that the blind learner is going to be defective in the interpretation of spatial and other perceptual terms (a hypothesis specifically countermanded by the findings of Landau et al., 1981, 1984); and that Kelli could not learn about the active/stative distinction (a hypothesis specifically countermanded by Experiment 4.5). This evidence aside, one is hard put to understand what this author believes could be *sensorily* available to any child—blind or sighted—to form the active/stative dichotomy. We hope that the evidence we have presented makes clear that opinions about what the blind can achieve, and opinions about how language is learned from the exposure conditions, require empirical defense.

4. We thank Elizabeth Shipley for discussion in which she suggested this solution to us.

5. Of course we do not mean to suggest that *blue* and *green* are "unnatural" in the sense that *grue* and *bleen* (cf. Goodman, 1979) surely are. Rather, *blue* and *green* are somewhat less natural than, say, *dog* or even *hot*, according to the criteria we are considering. Perhaps there is a continuum of relative naturalness.

6. We thank Eric Wanner for discussion in which he formulated the issues concerning relative binary contrasts as we have just described them.

7. It might seem that the claim for a simple binary opposition is too strong, given the existence of terms such as *medium, average, normal,* and *standard.* But notice that these are not the kind of frequent word that is in the vocabulary of two- and three-year-olds. More important, these are not dimensional terms like *big/small, deep/shallow,* but rather are general terms that apply across domains. (We thank Elizabeth Shipley for bringing this fact to our attention.) Thus there is extreme poverty in monomorphemic expressions for the midpoint on a specific dimension. One has to use constructive expressions (*midsized, middle-aged*) or general terms (*medium*) instead. In contrast, there are literally scores of relative polar pairs for specific spatial, locative, rate, temporal, mental-state dimensions, etc., and even adventitious (*clean/dirty*) dimensions. We should also point out that there are many crucial issues in understanding the use of the binary relative adjectives that we will not take up, for we have no special insight as to how they are to be described or explained. Chief among these is an explanation of the fact that usage of such adjectives *is* always domain-specific, in the sense that "big mouse" means 'big, for a mouse' and "small elephant" means 'small, for an elephant,' and hence a big mouse can be and always is smaller than a small elephant. It is rather surprising on the face of it that this seems to pose no problem to two- and three-year-old humans (see J. Katz, 1974, for an interesting discussion of the issues here, based on an analysis of the term *good*).

8. It is worth noting that this warm/cool distinction is made by Kay and McDaniel in a revision of Berlin and Kay's description of cross-linguistic color terms. The original distinction made by the latter authors—

black/white as the first cut made by a language evolving a color terminology—fails for both adult terminology and for the acquisition of color terms by the child.

9. We thank Elissa Newport for discussion in which she formulated the issue in this way.

10. For our simple example of *bat*, the likely answer presumably has to do with the unnatural yoking of inanimate and animate objects (cf. Keil, 1979). On the other hand, this line is blandly crossed for sponges as well as for toy dogs, so maybe the answer isn't as simple as it seems.

References

Abravanel, E. 1968. The development of intersensory patterning with regards to selected spatial dimensions. *Monographs of the Society for Research in Child Development* 33(2).

——— 1970. Choice for shape vs textural matching by young children. *Perceptual and Motor Skills* 31:527–533.

——— 1972. Short term memory for shape information processed intra and inter modally at three ages. *Perceptual and Motor Skills* 35:419–425.

Adelson, E. 1983. Precursors of early language development. In A. E. Mills, ed. *Language acquisition and the blind child.* London: Croom Helm.

Andersen, E., A. Dunlea, and L. Kekelis. 1984. Blind children's language: resolving some differences. *Journal of Child Language* 11(3):645–664.

Armstrong, J. D. 1978. The development of tactual maps. In G. Gordon, ed. *Active touch: The mechanism of recognition of objects by manipulation.* New York: Pergamon Press.

Armstrong, S., L. R. Gleitman, and H. Gleitman. 1983. What some concepts might not be. *Cognition* 13(3):263–308.

Bartlett, E. J. 1977. The acquisition of the meaning of color terms: A study of lexical development. In P. Smith and R. Campbell, eds. *Proceedings of the Sterling Conference on the psychology of language.* New York: Plenum Press.

Bates, E., and B. MacWhinney. 1982. Functionalist approaches to grammar. In E. Wanner and L. R. Gleitman, eds. *Language acquisition: State of the art.* New York: Cambridge University Press.

Bellugi, U. 1967. The acquisition of negation. Ph.D. diss., Harvard University.

Berkeley, G. 1709. An essay towards a new theory of vision. In D. M. Armstrong, ed. *Berkeley's philosophical writings.* New York: Macmillan, 1965.

Berla, E. P. 1982. Haptic perception of tangible graphic displays. In W. Schiff and E. Foulke, eds. *Tactual perception: A source book.* New York: Cambridge University Press.

Berlin, B., D. E. Breedlove, and P. H. Raven. 1974. *Principles of Tzeltal plant classification.* New York: Academic Press.

———— and P. Kay. 1969. *Basic color terms: Their universality and evolution.* Los Angeles: University of California Press.

Bever, T. G. 1970. The cognitive basis for linguistic structures. In J. Hayes, ed. *Cognition and the development of language.* New York: Wiley.

———— and P. S. Rosenbaum. 1970. Some lexical structures and their empirical validity. In R. A. Jacobs and P. S. Rosenbaum, eds. *Readings in English transformational grammar.* Waltham, Mass.: Ginn.

Bickerton, D. 1984. The language bioprogram hypothesis. *The Behavioral and Brain Sciences* 7(2):173–188.

Bierwisch, M. 1967. Some semantic universals of German adjectivals. *Foundations of Language* 3:1–36.

Bigelow, A. E. 1982. Early words of blind children. Paper presented at Canadian Psychological Association, Montreal.

———— 1983. Development of the use of sound in the search behavior of infants. *Developmental Psychology* 19:317–321.

———— 1984. The development of blind infants' search for dropped objects. Paper presented at International Conference on Infant Studies, New York.

Billman, D. 1983. Procedures for learning syntactic categories: A model and test with artificial grammars. Ph.D. diss., University of Michigan.

Blasdell, R., and P. Jensen. 1970. Stress and word position as determinants of imitation in first language learners. *Journal of Speech and Hearing Research* 13:193–202.

Bloom, L. 1970. *Language development: Form and function in emerging grammars.* Cambridge: MIT Press.

———— 1973. *One word at a time.* The Hague: Mouton.

———— 1983. Tensions in psycholinguistics. *Science* 220:843–844.

———— P. Lightbown, and L. Hood. 1975. Structure and variation in child language. *Monographs of the Society for Research in Child Development* 160.

Bolinger, D. 1977. Neutrality, norm, and bias. Manuscript.

Bloomfield, L. 1933. *Language.* New York: Holt.

Bornstein, M. H. 1975. Qualities of color vision in infancy. *Journal of Experimental Child Psychology* 19:401–419.

———— 1978. Chromatic vision in infancy. In H. Reese and L. Lipsitt, eds. *Advances in child development and behavior,* vol. 12. New York: Academic Press.

———— W. Kessen, and S. Weiskopf. 1976. Color vision and hue categorization in young human infants. *Journal of Experimental Psychology: Human Perception and Performance* 2:115–129.

Braine, M. D. S., and J. A. Hardy. 1982. On what case categories there are, why they are, and how they develop: An amalgam of *a priori* considerations, speculations, and evidence from children. In E. Wanner and L. R. Gleitman, eds. *Language acquisition: State of the art.* New York: Cambridge University Press.

Bresnan, J. 1978. A realistic transformational grammar. In M. Halle, J. Bresnan, and G. A. Miller, eds. *Linguistic theory and psychological reality.* Cambridge: MIT Press.

Brown, R. 1957. Linguistic determinism and parts of speech. *Journal of Abnormal and Social Psychology* 55:1–5.

———— 1973. *A first language.* Cambridge: Harvard University Press.

Bruner, J. S. 1974–75. From communication to language: A psychological perspective. *Cognition* 3:255–287.

Burlingham, D. 1964. Hearing and its role in the development of the blind. *The Psychoanalytic Study of the Child* 19:95–112.

Butterworth, G. 1983. Structure of the mind in human infancy. In L. Lipsitt, ed. *Advances in Infancy Research,* vol. 2. New Brunswick, N.J.: Ablex Corp.

Carey, S. 1982. Semantic development: The state of the art. In E. Wanner and L. R. Gleitman, eds. *Language acquisition: The state of the art.* New York: Cambridge University Press.

———— Forthcoming. *Conceptual Change in Childhood.* Cambridge: MIT Press, Bradford Books.

———— and E. J. Bartlett. 1978. Acquiring a single new word. *Papers and Reports on Child Language Development,* Department of Linguistics, Stanford University, 15:17–29.

Chi, M.T.H. 1978. Knowledge structures and memory development. In R. Siegler, ed. *Children's thinking: What develops?* Hillsdale: Erlbaum.

Chomsky, C. 1984. From hand to mouth: A study of speech and language through touch. Manuscript.

Chomsky, N. 1972. Some empirical issues in the theory of transformational grammar. In S. Peters, ed. *Goals of linguistic theory.* Englewood Cliffs, N.J.: Prentice-Hall.

———— 1975. *Reflections on language.* New York: Random House.

———— 1980. *Rules and representations.* New York: Columbia University Press.

Clark, E. V. 1973. What's in a word? On the child's acquisition of semantics in his first language. In T. Moore, ed. *Cognitive development and the acquisition of language.* New York: Academic Press.

Clark, H. H. 1973. Space, time, semantics, and the child. In T. Moore, ed. *Cognitive development and the acquisition of language.* New York: Academic Press.

Collis, G. M. 1977. Visual coordination and maternal speech. In H. R. Schaffer, *Studies in mother-infant interaction.* London: Academic Press.

Cooper, W. E., and J. Paccia-Cooper. 1980. *Syntax and speech.* Cambridge: Harvard University Press.

Cutsforth, T. D. 1951. *The blind in school and society.* New York: American Foundation for the Blind.

Darwin, C. H. 1877. A biographical sketch of a young child. *Kosmos,* 1:367–376 (as cited in Bornstein, 1978).

DeBoysson-Bardies, B., L. Sagart, and C. Durand. 1984. Discernible differences in the babbling of infants according to target language. *Journal of Child Language* 11:1–15.

DeVilliers, J. G., and P. A. DeVilliers. 1972. Early judgments of semantic and syntactic acceptability by children. *Journal of Psycholinguistic Research* 1:299–310.

Diamond, I. M. 1966. Zoological classification system of a primitive people. *Science* 151:1102–1104.

Dodd, C., and M. Lewis. 1969. The magnitude of the orienting response in children as a function of changes in color and contour. *Journal of Experimental Child Psychology* 8:269–305.

Dorian, N. 1978. The fate of morphological complexity in language death. *Language* 54(3):590–609.

Feldman, H., S. Goldin-Meadow, and L. R. Gleitman. 1978. Beyond Herodotus: The creation of language by linguistically deprived deaf children. In A. Lock, ed. *Action, symbol, and gesture: The emergence of language*. New York: Academic Press.

Fernald, A. 1982. Acoustic determinants of infant preference for "Motherese." Ph.D. diss., University of Oregon.

———— 1984. The perceptual and affective salience of mothers' speech to infants. In L. Feagans, C. Garvey, and R. Golinkoff, eds. *The origins and growth of communication*. New Brunswick, N.J.: Ablex Corp.

———— and T. Simon. 1984. Expanded intonation contours in mothers' speech to newborns. *Developmental Psychology* 20(1):104–113.

Fillmore, C. J. 1968. The case for case. In E. Bach and R. J. Harms, eds. *Universals in linguistic theory*. New York: Holt, Rinehart and Winston.

Flavell, J. H. 1977. The development of knowledge about visual perception. In *Nebraska Symposium on Motivation*, vol. 25. Lincoln: University of Nebraska Press.

Fodor, J. 1981. *Representations*. Cambridge: MIT Press, Bradford Books.

———— 1983. *The modularity of mind*. Cambridge: MIT Press, Bradford Books.

———— M. F. Garrett, E. T. Walker, and C. Parkes. 1980. Against definitions. *Cognition* 8(3):1–105.

Fodor, J. D., J. A. Fodor, and M. F. Garrett. 1975. The psychological unreality of semantic representations. *Linguistic Inquiry* 6(4):515–553.

Fraiberg, S. 1977. *Insights from the blind*. New York: Basic Books.

Freedman, D. A., B. J. Fox-Kolenda, D. A. Margileth, and D. H. Miller. 1969. The development of the use of sound as a guide to affective and cognitive behavior: A two-phase process. *Child Development* 40:1099–1105.

Furrow, D., K. Nelson, and H. Benedict. 1979. Mothers' speech to children and syntactic development: Some simple relationships. *Journal of Child Language* 6:423–442.

Garrett, M. F. 1975. The analysis of sentence production. In G. H. Bower, ed. *The psychology of learning and motivation*, vol. 9. New York: Academic Press.

Gentner, D. 1978. On relational meaning: The acquisition of verb meaning. *Child Development* 49:988–98.

———— 1982. Why nouns are learned before verbs: Linguistic relativity vs. natural partitioning. In S. Kuczaj, ed. *Language development: Language, culture, and cognition.* Hillsdale, N.J.: Erlbaum.

Gibson, E. J., and E. Spelke. 1983. The development of perception. In J. H. Flavell and E. Markman, eds. *Cognitive Development.* Vol. 3 of P. H. Mussen, ed. *Handbook of cognitive psychology.* New York: Wiley.

——— and A. S. Walker, 1984. Development of knowledge of visual-tactual affordances of substance. *Child Development* 55:453–460.

Gibson, J. J. 1979. *The ecological approach to visual perception.* Boston: Houghton Mifflin.

Givón, T. 1970. Notes on the semantic structure of English adjectives. *Language* 46:816–837.

Gleitman H. and L. R. Gleitman. 1979. Language use and language judgment. In C. J. Fillmore, D. Kempler, and W. S. Wang, eds. *Individual differences in language ability and language behavior.* New York: Academic Press.

Gleitman, L. R. 1965. Coordinating conjunctions in English. *Language* 41:260–293.

——— and H. Gleitman. 1970. *Phrase and paraphrase.* New York: Norton.

——— H. Gleitman, and E. F. Shipley. 1972. The emergence of the child as grammarian. *Cognition* 1(2):137–164.

——— and B. Landau. Forthcoming. The effect of gestational age at birth on the emergence of language.

——— E. L. Newport and H. Gleitman, 1984. The current status of the motherese hypothesis. *Journal of Child Language* 11(1):43–80.

——— and E. Wanner. 1982. Language acquisition: The state of the state of the art. In E. Wanner and L. R. Gleitman, eds. *Language acquisition: State of the art.* New York: Cambridge University Press.

——— and E. Wanner. 1984. Current issues in language learning. In M. H. Bornstein and M. E. Lamb, eds. *Developmental psychology: An advanced textbook.* Hillsdale, N.J.: Erlbaum.

Goldin-Meadow, S. 1982. The resilience of recursion: A study of a communication system developed without a conventional language model. In E. Wanner and L. R. Gleitman, eds. *Language acquisition: The state of the art.* New York: Cambridge University Press.

——— M. E. P. Seligman, and R. Gelman. 1976. Language in the two-year-old. *Cognition* 4(2):189–202.

Goodman, N. 1966. *The structure of appearance,* 2nd ed. Indianapolis, Ind.: Bobbs-Merrill.

——— *Fact, fiction and forecast.* 1979. Indianapolis, Ind.: Hackett.

Gordon, G., ed. 1978. *Active touch: The mechanism of recognition of objects by manipulation.* New York: Pergammon Press.

Gottfried, A. W., S. A. Rose, and W. H. Bridger. 1977. Cross-modal transfer in human infants. *Child Development* 48:118–123.

Grice, H. 1975. Logic and conversation. In P. Cole and J. L. Morgan, eds. *Syntax and semantics.* New York: Academic Press.

Grimshaw, J. 1983. Subcategorization and grammatical relations. In

A. Zaenen, ed. *Subjects and other subjects.* Evanston: Indiana University Linguistics Club.

Gruber, J. 1968 Look and see. *Language* 43:937–947.

Haith, M. M. 1980. *Rules that babies look by.* Hillsdale, N.J.: Erlbaum.

Harris, Z. S. 1951. *Methods in structural linguistics.* Chicago: University of Chicago Press.

Heider, E. 1972. "Focal" color areas and the development of color names. *Developmental Psychology* 4:447–455.

———— and D. Olivier. 1972. The structure of the color space in naming and memory for two languages. *Cognitive Psychology* 3:337–354.

Hermelin, B., and N. O'Connor. 1982. Spatial modality coding in children with and without impairments. In M. Potegal, ed. *Spatial abilities: Development and physiological foundations.* New York: Academic Press.

Hirsch-Pasek, K., L. R. Gleitman, and H. Gleitman. 1978. What did the brain say to the mind? A study of the detection and report of ambiguity by young children. In A. Sinclair, R. J. Jarvella, and W. J. M. Levelt, eds. *The child's conception of language.* Berlin: Springer-Verlag.

Hochberg, J. *Perception.* Englewood Cliffs, N.J.: Prentice-Hall, 1978.

Hofsten, C. von. 1982. Eye-hand coordination in the newborn. *Developmental Psychology* 18:450–456.

Hume, D. 1758. *An inquiry concerning human understanding.* Indianapolis, Ind.: Bobbs-Merrill, 1955.

Huttenlocher, J. S., P. Smiley, and R. Charney. 1983. Emergence of action categories in the child: Evidence from verb meanings. *Psychological Review* 90:(1):72–93.

Isotomina, Z. M. 1963. Perception and naming of color in early childhood. *Soviet Journal of Psychiatry* 1(2):37–45.

Jackendoff, R. 1972. *Semantic interpretation in generative grammar.* Cambridge: MIT Press.

———— 1976. Toward an explanatory semantic representation, *Linguistic Inquiry* 7(1): 89–150.

———— 1983. *Semantics and cognition.* Cambridge: MIT Press.

Jakobson, R. 1939. *Selected writings.* The Hague: Mouton.

Johansson, L. 1984. Mothers' descriptions of parts and wholes to young children. Manuscript, Columbia University.

Jones, B. 1972. Development of cutaneous and kinesthetic localization by blind and sighted children. *Developmental Psychology* 6:349–352.

———— 1975. Spatial perception in the blind. *British Journal of Psychology* 66:461–472.

Joshi, A. 1975. Factorization of verbs. In C. H. Heidrick, ed. *Semantics and communication.* Amsterdam: North Holland.

Katz, J. J. 1964. Semantic theory and the meaning of good. *Journal of Philosophy* 61(23):739–766.

———— 1972. *Semantic theory.* Cambridge: MIT Press.

———— and J. A. Fodor. 1963. The structure of a semantic theory. *Language* 39:170–210.

Katz, N., E. Baker, and J. MacNamara. 1974. What's in a name? A study of how children learn common and proper names. *Child Development* 45:469–473.

Kay, P., and C. K. McDaniel. 1978. The linguistic significance of the meanings of basic color terms. *Language* 54(3):610–646.

Kean, M. L. 1979. Agrammatism: A phonological deficit? *Cognition* 7(1):69–84.

Keil, F. C. 1979. *Semantic and conceptual development.* Cambridge: Harvard University Press.

—— and N. Batterman. 1984. A characteristic-to-defining shift in the development of word meaning. *Journal of Verbal Learning and Verbal Behavior* 23(2): 221–236.

Kekelis, L., and E. Andersen. 1984. Family communication styles and language development. *Journal of Visual Impairment and Blindness.* Feb.: 54–65.

Kemler, D. J. 1983. Holistic and analytic modes in perceptual and cognitive development. In T. Tighe and B. E. Shepp, eds. *Perception, cognition, and development: Interactional analyses.* Hillsdale, N.J.: Erlbaum.

Kennedy, J. 1978. Haptics. In E. Carterette and M. P. Friedman, eds. *Handbook of perception,* vol. 8. New York: Academic Press.

Klatt, D. H. 1975. Vowel lengthening is syntactically determined in a connected discourse. *Journal of Phonetics* 3:229–240.

—— 1976. Linguistic uses of segmental duration in English: Acoustic and perceptual evidence. *Journal of the Acoustic Society of America* 59:1208–1221.

Kripke, S. 1977. *Naming, necessity, and natural kinds.* Ithaca, N.Y.: Cornell University Press.

Ladefoged, P. 1975. *A course in phonetics.* New York: Harcourt Brace Jovanivich.

Landau, B. 1982a. Will the real grandmother please stand up? *Journal of Psycholinguistic Research* 11(2):47–62.

—— 1982b. Language learning in blind children. Ph.D. diss., University of Pennsylvania.

—— 1984. Early map use by a congenitally blind child. Manuscript.

—— H. Gleitman, and E. S. Spelke. 1981. Spatial knowledge and geometric representation in a child blind from birth. *Science* 213:1275–1278.

—— E. S. Spelke, and H. Gleitman. 1984b. Spatial knowledge in a young blind child. *Cognition* 16(3):225–260.

Lederman, S. J. 1978. Heightening tactile impressions of surface texture. In G. Gordon, ed. *Active touch: The mechanism of recognition of objects by manipulation.* New York: Pergammon Press.

Lempers, J. D., E. R. Flavell, and J. H. Flavell. 1977. The development in very young children of tacit knowledge concerning visual perception. *Genetic Psychology Monographs* 95:3–53.

Lenneberg, E. H. 1967. *Biological Foundations of Language.* New York: Wiley.

Leonard, J. A., and R. C. Newman. 1967. Spatial orientation in the blind. *Nature* 215:1413–1414.

Levy, Y. 1983a. It's frogs all the way down. *Cognition* 15:75–93.

———— 1983b. The acquisition of Hebrew plurals: The case of the missing gender category. *Journal of Child Language* 10:107–121.

Lewis, M., and M. H. Baumel, 1970. A study in the orienting of attention. *Perceptual and Motor Skills* 31:979–990.

Liberman, M., and L. Streeter. 1976. Use of nonsense syllable mimicry in the study of prosodic phenomena. Paper delivered at Acoustical Society of America meeting, San Diego (as cited in Liberman and Prince, 1977).

———— and A. Prince. 1977. On stress and linguistic rhythm. *Linguistic Inquiry* 8(2):249–336.

Locke, J. 1690. *An essay concerning human understanding.* A. D. Woozley, ed. Cleveland: Meridian Books, 1964.

Maratsos, M. 1982. The child's construction of grammatical categories. In E. Wanner and L. R. Gleitman, eds. *Language acquisition: The state of the art.* New York: Cambridge University Press.

———— and M. A. Chalkley. 1980. The internal language of children's syntax: The ontogenesis and representation of syntactic categories. In K. Nelson, ed. *Children's language,* vol. 2. New York: Gardner Press.

Markman, E. M., and J. E. Hutchinson. 1984. Children's sensitivity to constraints on word meaning: Taxonomic versus thematic relations. *Cognitive Psychology* 16(1):1–27.

Marmor, G. S. 1978. Age of onset of blindness and the development of the semantics of color names. *Journal of Experimental Child Psychology* 00:267–277.

Marin, O., E. Saffran, and M. Schwartz. 1976. Dissociations of language in aphasia: Implications for normal function. *Annals of the New York Academy of Sciences,* 280:863–884.

Masur, E. F. 1982. Mothers' responses to infants' object-related gestures: Influences on lexical development. *Journal of Child Language* 9(1):23–30.

McCawley, J. D. 1970. Where do noun phrases come from? In R. A. Jacobs and P. S. Rosenbaum, eds. *Readings in English transformational grammar.* Waltham, Mass.: Ginn.

McNeill, D. 1966. The creation of language by children. In J. Lyons and R. Wales, eds. *Psycholinguistics papers.* Edinburgh: Edinburgh University Press.

Mervis, C. B., and M. Crisafi, 1978. Order of acquisition of subordinate, basic, and superordinate level categories. *Child Development* 49(4):988–998.

———— and J. R. Pani. 1980. Acquisition of basic object categories. *Cognitive Psychology* 12:496–522.

Millar, S. 1974. Tactile short-term memory by blind and sighted children. *British Journal of Psychology* 65:(2):253–263.

———— 1978. Aspects of memory for information from touch and movement, in G. Gordon, ed. *Active touch: The mechanism of recognition of objects by manipulation.* New York: Pergammon Press.

Miller, G., and P. Johnson-Laird. 1976. *Language and perception*. Cambridge: Harvard University Press.

Mithun, M. 1982. The acquisition of polysynthesis. Manuscript (cited in A. Peters, 1984).

Mulford, R. In press. First words of the blind child. In M. D. Smith and J. L. Locke, eds. *The emergent lexicon: The child's development of a linguistic vocabulary*. New York: Academic Press.

Nakatani, L., and K. Dukes. 1977. Locus of segmental cues for word juncture. *Journal of the Acoustic Society of America* 62(3):714–724.

——— and J. Schaffer. 1978. Hearing "words" without words: Prosodic cues for word perception. *Journal of the Acoustic Society of America* 63(1):234–245.

Nelson, K. 1973. Structure and strategy in learning to talk. *Monograph of the Society for Research in Child Development* 38(1–2).

——— 1974. Concept, word, and sentence: Intercorrelations in acquisition and development. *Psychological Review* 81:267–285.

Newport, E. L. 1977. Motherese: The speech of mothers to young children. In N. Castellan, D. Pisoni, and G. Potts, eds. *Cognitive theory*, vol. 2. Hillsdale, N.J.: Erlbaum.

——— 1982. Task specificity in language learning? Evidence from speech perception and American Sign Language. In E. Wanner and L. R. Gleitman, eds. *Language acquisition: The state of the art*. New York: Cambridge University Press.

——— 1984. Constraints on learning: Studies in the acquisition of American Sign Language. *Papers and Reports on Child Language Development*, 23 (Stanford University), pp. 1–22.

——— H. Gleitman, and L. R. Gleitman. 1977. Mother, I'd rather do it myself: Some effects and non-effects of maternal speech style. In C. E. Snow and C. A. Ferguson, eds. *Talking to children: Language input and acquisition*. New York: Cambridge University Press.

——— and R. P. Meier. In press. Acquisition of American Sign Language. In D. I. Slobin, ed. *The cross-linguistic study of language acquisition*. Hillsdale, N.J.: Erlbaum.

——— and T. Supalla. In progress. Critical period effects in the acquisition of a primary language.

Ninio. A. 1980. Ostensive definition in vocabulary teaching. *Journal of Child Language* 7(3):565–574.

——— and J. Bruner. 1978. The achievement and antecedents of labelling. *Journal of Child Language.* 5:1–15.

Norris, M., P. J. Spaulding, and F. H. Brodie. 1957. *Blindness in Children.* Chicago: University of Chicago Press.

Osherson, D. 1978. Three conditions on conceptual naturalness. *Cognition* 6(4):263–290.

Park, S., K. Tsukagoshi, and B. Landau. 1984. Children's mis-naming of colors: An hypothesis and some evidence from English and Japanese. Manuscript.

Peters, A. 1984. Speech delivered at the Graduate School of Education, University of Pennsylvania.

Piaget, J. 1954. *The construction of reality in the child.* New York: Basic Books.

—— and B. Inhelder. 1948. *The child's conception of space.* New York: Norton, 1967.

Pinker, S. 1982. A theory of the acquisition of lexical interpretive grammars. In J. Bresnan, ed. *The mental representation of grammatical relations.* Cambridge: MIT Press.

—— 1984. *Language learnability and language development.* Cambridge: Harvard University Press.

Putnam, H. 1975. The meaning of 'meaning.' In H. Putnam, *Mind, language, and reality: Philosophical papers,* vol. 2. New York: Cambridge University Press.

Pye. C. 1983. Mayan telegraphese. *Language* 59(3):583–604.

Quine, W. V. 1960. *Word and object.* Cambridge: MIT Press.

Read, C., and P. Schreiber. 1982. Why short subjects are harder to find than long ones. In E. Wanner and L. R. Gleitman, eds. *Language acquisition: State of the art.* New York: Cambridge University Press.

Rescorla, L. 1980. Overextension in early language development. *Journal of Child Language* 7(2):321–336.

Rice, M. 1980. *Cognition to language: Categories, word meanings, and training.* Baltimore: University Park Press.

Rosch, E. 1973. On the internal structure of perceptual and semantic categories. In T. E. Moore, ed. *Cognitive development and the acquisition of language.* New York: Academic Press.

—— 1978. Principles of categorization. In E. Rosch and B. Lloyd, eds. *Cognition and categorization.* Hillsdale, N.J.: Erlbaum.

—— C. B. Mervis, W. D. Gray, D. M. Johnson, and P. Boyes-Braem. 1976. Basic objects in natural categories. *Cognitive Psychology* 8:382–439.

Rose, S. A., M. S. Blank, and W. Bridger. 1972. Intermodal and intramodal retention of visual and tactual information in young children. *Developmental Psychology* 6(3):482–486.

—— A. W. Gottfried, and W. H. Bridger. 1981. Cross-modal transfer in six-month-old infants. *Developmental Psychology* 17(5):661–669.

Rozin, P., and L. R. Gleitman. 1977. The structure and acquisition of reading, II: The reading process and the acquisition of the alphabetic principle. In A. S. Reber and D. Scarborough, eds. *Toward a psychology of reading.* Hillsdale, N.J.: Erlbaum.

Ruff, H. 1984. Infants' manipulative exploration of objects: Effects of age and object characteristics. *Developmental Psychology* 20(1):9–20.

Sankoff, G., and S. LaBerge. 1973. On the acquisition of native speakers by a language. *Kivung* 6:32–47.

Schaffer, R. 1977. *Mothering.* Cambridge: Harvard University Press.

Schieffelin, B. B. *How Kaluli children learn what to say, what to do, and how to feel: An ethnographic study of the development of communicative competence.* New York: Cambridge University Press, 1982.

Schiff, W., and E. Foulke, eds. *Tactual perception: A sourcebook.* New York: Cambridge University Press, 1982.

Schlesinger, I. M. 1971. The production of utterances and language acquisition. In D. I. Slobin, ed. *The ontogenesis of grammar: A theoretical symposium.* New York: Academic Press.

Searle, J. R. 1975. Indirect speech acts. In P. Cole and J. Morgan, eds. *Syntax and semantics: Speech acts.* New York: Academic Press.

Shatz, M. 1982. On mechanisms of language acquisition: Can features of the communicative environment account for development. In E. Wanner and L. R. Gleitman, eds. *Language acquisition: State of the art.* New York: Cambridge University Press.

Shipley, E. F., and I. F. Kuhn. 1983. A constraint on comparisons: Equally detailed alternatives. *Journal of Experimental Child Psychology* 35:195–222.

——— I. F. Kuhn, and E. C. Madden. 1983. Mothers' use of superordinate terms. *Journal of Child Language* 10(3):571–588.

——— C. S. Smith, and L. R. Gleitman. 1969. A study in the acquisition of language: Free responses to commands. *Language* 45:322–342.

Slobin, D. I. 1966. Grammatical transformations and sentence comprehension in childhood and adulthood. *Journal of Verbal Learning and Verbal Behavior* 5:219–227.

——— 1973. Cognitive prerequisites for the development of grammar. In C. A. Ferguson and D. I. Slobin, eds. *Studies of child language development.* New York: Holt, Rinehart, and Winston.

——— 1981. The origins of grammatical encoding of events. In W. Deutsch, ed. *The child's construction of language.* New York: Academic Press.

——— 1982. Universal and particular in the acquisition of language. In E. Wanner and L. R. Gleitman, eds. *Language acquisition: The state of the art.* New York: Cambridge University Press.

Smith, E. E., and D. L. Medin. 1981. *Categories and concepts.* Cambridge: Harvard University Press.

Smith, L. B., and D. G. Kemler. 1977. Developmental trends in free classification: Evidence for a new conceptualization of perceptual development. *Journal of Experimental Child Psychology* 24:279–298.

Snow, C. E. 1977. Mothers' speech research: From input to interaction. In C. E. Snow and C. A. Ferguson, eds. *Talking to children: Language input and acquisition.* New York: Cambridge University Press.

Sommers, F. 1959. The ordinary language tree. *Mind* 68:160–185.

Spelke, E. S. 1979. Perceiving bimodally specified events in infancy. *Developmental Psychology* 15:626–636.

——— 1982. Perceptual knowledge of objects in infancy. In J. Mehler, E. C. T. Walker, and M. Garrett, eds. *Perspectives on mental representations.* Hillsdale, N.J.: Erlbaum.

Spring, D. R., and P. S. Dale. 1977. Discrimination of linguistic stress in early infancy. *Journal of Speech and Hearing Research* 20:224–231.

Streeter, L. A. 1978. Acoustic determinants of phrase boundary perception. *Journal of the Acoustic Society of America* 64:1582–1592.

Sullivan, E. V., and M. T. Turvey. 1972. Short-term retention of tactile stimulation. *Quarterly Journal of Experimental Psychology* 24:253–261.

Supalla, T. In press. *Structure and acquisition of verbs of motion and location in American Sign Language.* Cambridge: MIT Press, Bradford Books.

Talmy, L. 1983. How language structures space. In H. Pick and L. Acredolo, eds. *Spatial orientation: Theory, research, and application.* New York: Plenum Press.

Tetzchner, S. von, and H. Maitinsen. 1980. A psycholinguistic study of the language of the blind, I: Verbalism. *International Journal of Psycholinguistics* 1–3(19):49–61.

Thomson, J., and R. Chapman. 1976. Who is "daddy" revisited: The status of 2-year-olds' over-extended words in use and comprehension. *Journal of Child Language.* 4:359–375.

Tversky, A. 1977. Features of similarity. *Psychological Review,* 84(4):327–352.

———— and I. Gati. 1978. Studies of similarity. In E. Rosch and B. Lloyd, eds. *Cognition and categorization.* Hillsdale, N.J.: Erlbaum.

Urwin, C. 1983. Dialogue and cognitive functioning in the early language development of three blind children. In A. E. Mills, ed. *Language acquisition in the blind child.* London: Croom Helm.

Vendler, Z. 1972. *Res cogitans,* Ithaca, N.Y.: Cornell University Press.

Warren D. H. 1977. *Blindness and early childhood development.* New York: American Foundation for the Blind.

———— 1982. The development of haptic perception. In W. Schiff and E. Foulke, eds. *Tactual perception: A sourcebook.* New York: Cambridge University Press.

Waxman, S., and R. Gelman. 1984. Superordinate classification in preschool children. Manuscript.

Werth, P. 1983. Meaning in language acquisition. In A. E. Mills, ed. *Language acquisition in the blind child.* London: Croom Helm.

Wexler, K., and P. Culicover. 1980. *Formal principles of language acquisition.* Cambridge: MIT Press.

Whorf, B. 1956. *Language, thought, and reality* (J. Carroll, ed.). New York: Wiley.

Young-Browne, G., H. M. Rosenfeld and F. D. Horowitz. 1977. Infant discrimination of facial expression. *Child Development* 48:555–562.

Zaporozhets, A. V. 1965. The development of perception in the preschool child. In P. H. Mussen, ed. European research in cognitive development. *Monographs of the Society for Research in Child Development* 30:82–101.

Index